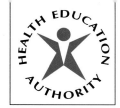

the Pregnancy book

Your complete guide
to pregnancy, childbirth
and the first few weeks
with a new baby

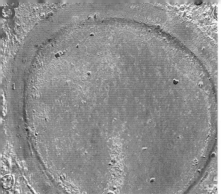

Contents

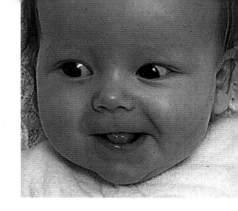

Your pregnancy at a glance

0-8 *weeks*

- Pregnancy test – you can have one from the first day of a missed period, if you wish (see **Finding out**, page 26).

- Make an early appointment to see your GP or a midwife if you know you're pregnant or think you may be (see **Finding out**, page 26). Begin to think about where you want your baby to be born (see **Deciding where to have your baby**, page 33). Ask about antenatal care (see **Antenatal care and antenatal classes**, page 51).

- Some mothers start to feel sick or tired around this time or have other minor physical problems for a few weeks (see **Common minor problems**, page 77).

- Take a folic acid supplement and try to eat a balanced diet (see pages 8-12).

8-12 *weeks*

- You'll probably attend your first antenatal appointment. Appointments will usually be monthly at first (see **Antenatal care and antenatal classes**, page 51).

- Ask about your rights at work and the benefits available (see **Rights and benefits**, page 133).

- If you're on Income Support or income-based Jobseeker's Allowance, you can claim free milk tokens (see **Rights and benefits**, page 133).

- Make a dental appointment. Dental care is free during pregnancy.

12-16 *weeks*

- Find out about antenatal classes if you have not already done so (see **Antenatal care and antenatal classes**, page 51).

- Begin to think about how you want to feed your baby (see **The feeding question**, page 66).

- Make sure you're wearing a bra which supports well.

- You may be offered an ultrasound scan which will show your baby moving. Your partner may like to see this too (see **Antenatal care and antenatal classes**, page 51).

- If you've been feeling sick and tired in the early weeks, you will probably start to feel better around this time.

- You may be offered tests to check for abnormalities in the baby (see pages 56-9).

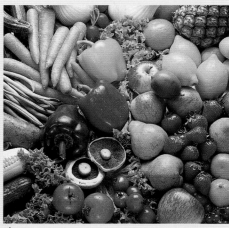

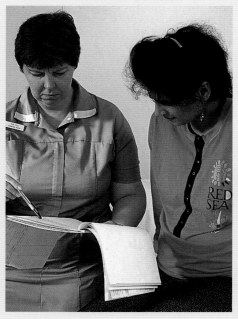

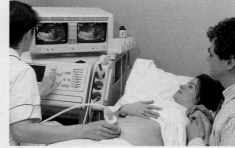

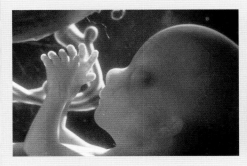
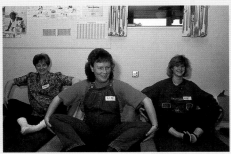
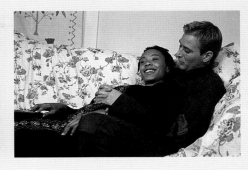

16-20 *weeks*

- You *may* start to feel your baby move (see **How the baby develops**, page 31).

- Your tummy will begin to get bigger and you'll need looser clothes.

- You may feel a new surge of energy around this time.

- Try to do your pregnancy exercises regularly (see **Your health in pregnancy**, page 16). Ask your doctor or midwife to let you hear your baby's heartbeat.

20-24 *weeks*

- Your womb will begin to enlarge more rapidly and you'll really begin to look pregnant.

- You may feel hungrier than before. Stick to a sensible balanced diet (see **Your health in pregnancy**, page 16).

- Make sure you've booked into antenatal classes if you wish to attend (see pages 64–5).

24-28 *weeks*

- Get your maternity certificate, form MAT B1, from your doctor or midwife (see **Rights and benefits**, pages 130–40).

- If you're taking maternity leave, inform your employer in writing *at least* three weeks before you stop work (see **Rights and benefits**, page 137).

- If you're claiming Statutory Maternity Pay (SMP), write to your employer at least three weeks before you stop work (see **Rights and benefits**, page 136).

- If you're claiming Maternity Allowance, do so as soon as you can after you are 26 weeks pregnant (see **Rights and benefits**, pages 133-5).

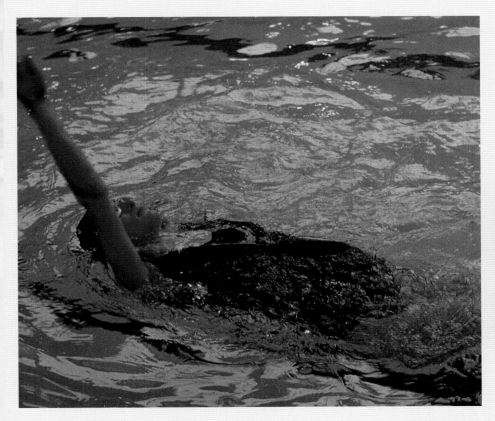

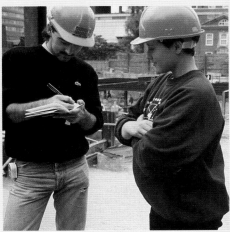

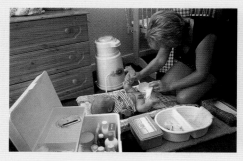
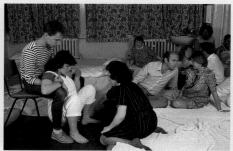
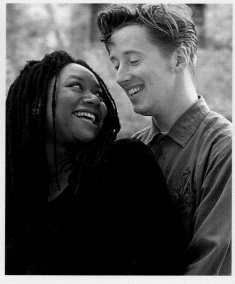

28-32 *weeks*

- If you're on Income Support, income-based Jobseeker's Allowance or Family Credit, you can claim a lump sum maternity payment to help buy things for your new baby (see **Rights and benefits**, pages 131-2).

- Think about what you need for the baby, if you have not already done so (see **What you need for the baby**, pages 85-8).

- If you have young children, spend time getting them used to the idea of a new baby.

- Check that your shoes are comfortable. If you get tired, try to rest with your feet above the level of your heart.

- You'll probably now attend for antenatal care every fortnight.

32-36 *weeks*

- Make arrangements for the birth, in hospital or at home. If you have children already, decide who will look after them.

- Pack your bag ready for the hospital, or make sure that you have been provided with a home delivery pack.

- You'll probably be attending antenatal classes now (see **Antenatal care and antenatal classes**, page 51).

- You may be more aware of your womb tightening from time to time. These are mild contractions (see **Labour and birth**, page 90).

- You may feel quite tired. Make sure you get plenty of rest.

36 *weeks onwards*

- You'll probably be attending antenatal care weekly until your baby is born.

- Make sure you have all important telephone numbers handy in case labour starts (see **Labour and birth**, page 89).

- The last few weeks can seem very long. Plan some interesting things to do to take your mind off waiting.

- Telephone your hospital or midwife if you have any worries about labour or the birth.

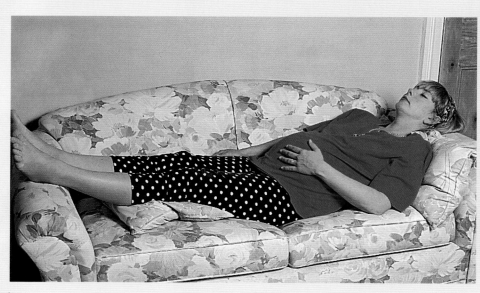
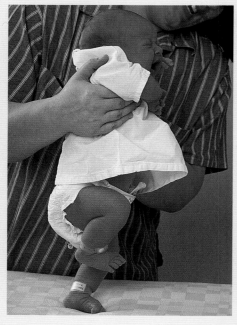

Introduction

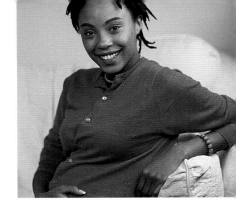

Every parent is different, just as every baby is different. So there can't be many rules to having a baby. But you will find a lot of information in these pages which should help you to decide what you will do, how you will cope and, most of all, how you can best enjoy both pregnancy and your baby.

Chapter 1 is about what you can do to make sure you and your baby stay healthy during your pregnancy. The book then takes you through pregnancy, birth and the first two weeks of caring for your baby. You may want to read some chapters several times, or look up specific things which interest or concern you. To find a topic quickly, just look at the index at the back of the book.

If there is anything which puzzles you, or if you need further explanation, don't hesitate to ask your doctor, midwife or health visitor.

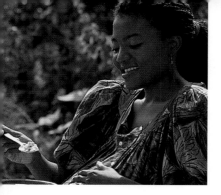

1 Your health in pregnancy

This chapter describes some of the things you should think about to make sure you and your baby stay healthy during pregnancy.

WHAT SHOULD YOU EAT?

A healthy diet is an important part of a healthy lifestyle at any time, but particularly if you are pregnant or are planning a pregnancy. Eating healthily during pregnancy will help your baby develop and grow and will help keep you fit and well. You don't need to go on a special diet, but make sure that you eat a variety of different foods every day in order to get the right balance of nutrients that you and your baby need. You should also avoid certain foods to be on the safe side.

There's no need to 'eat for two' when you are pregnant. It's the quality not the quantity that's important. With a few exceptions you can continue to eat all the foods you enjoy (see *Take care with some foods*, page 11). Eating healthily often means just changing the amounts of different foods that you eat rather than cutting out all your favourites. *The Balance of Good Health* illustrates the mixture of different foods you need in your diet and the proportions you should eat them in. This is illustrated below.

THE BALANCE OF GOOD HEALTH

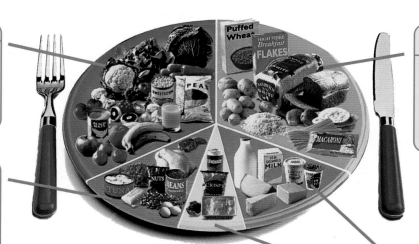

Fruit and vegetables

Try to eat at least five servings a day. This can include a glass of pure fruit juice. This food group includes fresh frozen and canned fruit and vegetables, salads, dried fruit, fruit juices.

Meat. fish and alternatives

Eat one or two servings a day. Choose lean meat, remove the skin from poultry and cook using the minimum of fat. Try to eat oily fish at least once a week. This food group includes meat (except liver), fish, poultry, eggs, beans, pulses, nuts (except peanuts).

Bread, other cereals and potatoes

Make these the main part of every meal, eat wholegrain varieties when you can. This food group includes bread, potatoes, breakfast cereals, pasta, rice, oats, noodles, maize, millet, yams, cornmeal, sweet potatoes.

Foods containing fat, foods containing sugar

Limit the amount you eat. This food group includes all spreading fats, oils, salad dressings, cream, chocolate, crisps, biscuits, pastries, ice-cream, cake, puddings, fizzy drinks.

Milk and dairy foods

Try to eat several servings a day, using low-fat varieties whenever you can. This food group includes milk, yoghurt, fromage frais.

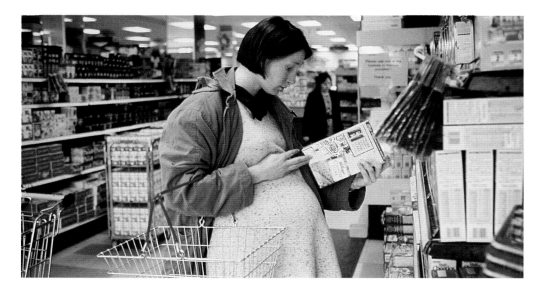

● **Eat plenty of fruit and vegetables** as these provide the vitamins and minerals, as well as fibre which helps digestion and prevents constipation. Eat them lightly cooked in a little water or raw to get the most out of them. Frozen, tinned and dried fruit and vegetables are good too.

● **Starchy foods like bread, potatoes, rice, pasta, chapatis, yams and breakfast cereals** are an important part of any diet and should, with vegetables, form the main part of any meal. They are satisfying, without containing too many calories, and are an important source of vitamins and fibre. Try eating wholemeal bread and wholegrain cereals when you can.

● **Lean meat, fish, poultry, eggs, cheese, beans and pulses** are all good sources of nutrients. Eat some every day.

● **Dairy foods, like milk, cheese and yoghurt** are important as they contain calcium and other nutrients needed for your baby's development. Choose low-fat varieties wherever possible. You can get seven pints of milk free per week if you are on income Support or income-based Jobseeker's Allowance (see page 133).

● **Try to cut down on sugar and sugary foods** like sweets, biscuits and cakes and sugary drinks like cola. Sugar contains calories without providing any other nutrients the body needs. It also adds to the risk of tooth decay.

● **Cut down on fat and fatty foods as well.** Most of us eat far more fat than we need. Fat is very high in calories and too much can cause excess weight gain and increase the risk of heart disease and it can contribute to being overweight. Avoid fried foods, trim the fat off meat, use spreads sparingly and go easy on foods like pastry, chocolate and chips which contain a lot of fat. Choose low-fat varieties of dairy products, for example semi-skimmed or skimmed milk, low-fat yoghurt and half-fat hard cheese.

Have drinks which contain caffeine – coffee, tea and colas – in moderation, as there may be a slight risk that too much caffeine will affect your baby's birthweight. Try decaffeinated tea and coffee, fruit juice or mineral water.

VITAMIN SUPPLEMENTS

It's best to get the vitamins and minerals you need from the food you eat. Some people, like those on a restricted diet, need extra, especially vitamin D. Ask your doctor whether you should take vitamin supplements. Don't take extra vitamin A supplements without advice as too much could harm your baby.

FOLIC ACID

This vitamin is special (see this page). You need to take a 400 microgram (0.4 milligram) tablet every day from the time you start trying to conceive. Continue taking the supplement right up until you're 12 weeks pregnant. Even if you didn't take folic acid before conceiving, it's worth starting as soon as you find out that you're pregnant and you should still continue until you're 12 weeks pregnant. If you have had a baby with spina bifida before, or are taking medication for epilepsy, you will need to take a bigger dose of folic acid. Speak to your doctor about this.

Foods carrying this mark have added folic acid.

VITAMINS AND MINERALS

- Green, leafy vegetables, lean meat, dried fruit and nuts (see page 12 on peanuts) contain **iron**. If you are short of iron you're likely to get very tired and may suffer from anaemia.

- Citrus fruit, tomatoes, broccoli, blackcurrants and potatoes are good sources of **vitamin C**, which you need to help you to absorb iron.

- Dairy products, fish with edible bones like sardines, bread, nuts (see page 12) and green vegetables are rich in **calcium**, which is vital for making bones and teeth.

- Margarine, oily fish (like sardines) and taramasalata contain **vitamin D** to keep your bones healthy and to provide your baby with vitamin D to last during the first few months of life. The best source of vitamin D is summer sunlight, but make sure that you wear a high protection sunblock when you are in the sunlight and never burn. If you have dark skin, or always cover your skin, you may be particularly at risk of vitamin D deficiency. Ask your doctor if you need to take a vitamin D supplement.

- You need extra **folic acid** from the time you start trying to conceive until the 12th week of pregnancy. This can help prevent birth defects, which are known as neural tube defects, such as spina bifida. You can get folic acid from green, leafy vegetables, but don't overcook them as this destroys the vitamin. Some breakfast cereals and breads have had folic acid added to them, so look at the label. Regardless of what you eat, always take a 400 microgram (0.4 milligram) folic acid tablet every day.

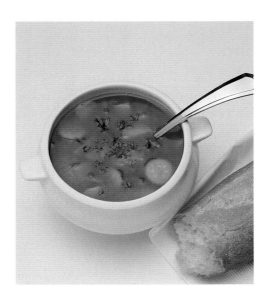

These are available from pharmacies and supermarkets or your GP may be able to prescribe them for you. Ask your GP or pharmacist for advice if you are unsure.

WELFARE FOOD SCHEME

If you receive Income Support or a Jobseeker's Allowance, you are entitled to:

- supplements of vitamins A, C and D;

- seven pints of cow's milk per week.

These are free to pregnant and breastfeeding mothers and supplements are available at very low cost to all mothers from maternity and child health clinics. For further information see leaflet *Welfare Milk and Vitamins – a guide for families* (WMV:G1) (in Northern Ireland see *Free milk and vitamins – a guide for families* WM V1 G1 (NI)), available from social security offices or the Benefits Agency.

VEGETARIAN, VEGAN AND SPECIAL DIETS

Providing a vegetarian diet is varied and balanced, it will provide adequate nutrients for you and your baby during pregnancy. However, iron and vitamin B12 can be hard to obtain from a vegetarian diet. Talk to your doctor or midwife about ways to increase intakes of these important nutrients. If you are vegan (i.e. you cut out all animal products from your diet), or you follow another type of restricted diet such as gluten free, for example, because of food intolerance e.g Coeliac disease or for religious reasons, talk to your doctor or midwife. Ask to be referred to a dietitian for advice on how to eat healthily during pregnancy.

HEALTHY SNACKS

- Sandwiches or pitta bread filled with grated cheese, lean ham, mashed tuna, salmon or sardines and salad

- Salad vegetables washed thoroughly

- Low-fat yoghurt and fromage frais

- Hummus and bread or vegetable sticks

- Ready-to-eat apricots, figs or prunes

- Vegetable and bean soups

- Unsweetened breakfast cereals or porridge and milk

- Milky drinks or unsweetened fruit juices

- Fresh fruit

- Baked beans on toast or baked potato

TAKE CARE WITH SOME FOODS

Besides eating a wide variety of foods, there are certain precautions you should take in order to safeguard your baby's well being as well as your own.

- **Cook all meat and poultry thoroughly** so that there is no trace of pink or blood and wash all surfaces and utensils after preparing raw meat. This will help to avoid infection with Toxoplasma, which may cause toxoplasmosis and can harm your baby (see page 18).

- **Wash fruit, vegetables and salads** to remove all traces of soil which may contain Toxoplasma.

- **Make sure eggs are thoroughly cooked** until the whites and yolks are solid, to prevent the risk of Salmonella food poisoning, and avoid foods containing raw and undercooked eggs like home-made mayonnaise, ice-cream, cheesecake or mousse.

- **Avoid eating all types of paté and mould-ripened soft cheese**, like Brie and Camembert, and similar blue-veined varieties, like Stilton or Danish blue, because of the risk of Listeria infection. You can eat hard cheeses such as cheddar and parmesan, and other cheeses made from pasteurised milk such as cottage cheese, mozzarella cheese and cheese spreads. Although Listeria is a very rare disease, it is important to take special precautions during pregnancy because even the mild form of the illness can lead to miscarriage, stillbirth or severe illness in the newborn.

> ## PREGNANCY AND WEIGHT
> *Most women gain between 10–12.5 kg (22–28 lb). Weight gain varies a great deal and depends on your weight before pregnancy. If you're concerned, talk to your midwife or GP. They may have special advice for you if you weigh more than 100 kg or less than 50 kg.*

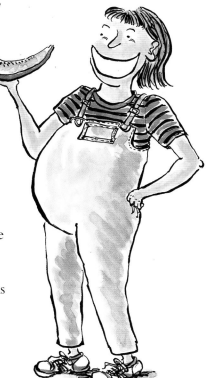

FURTHER READING

- Food safety *is available free from Foodsense London SE99 7TT tel. 0645 556 000.*

- While you are pregnant: how to avoid infection from food and contact with animals *is available free of charge from the Department of Health, PO Box 410, Wetherby LS23 7LN. (In Northern Ireland* While you are pregnant *is available from the Central Health Promotion Resource Service in your local Health and Social Services Board area)*

- Folic acid: what all women should know *is available free from your doctor or clinic. (In Northern Ireland ask for* Folic Acid: one of life's essentials*)*

- **Drink only pasteurised or UHT milk** which has had the harmful germs destroyed. If only raw or green-top milk is available, boil it before you drink it. Don't drink unpasteurised goat's or sheep's milk or eat their milk products.

- **Don't eat liver or liver products**, like liver paté or liver sausage, as they may contain a lot of vitamin A. Too much vitamin A could harm your baby.

- **Avoid eating peanuts and foods containing peanut products** (e.g. peanut butter, unrefined groundnut oil, some snacks, etc.) if you or your baby's father or any previous children have a history of hayfever, asthma, eczema or other allergies. This may reduce the risk of your baby developing a potentially serious allergy to peanuts. Read food labels carefully and, if you are still in doubt about the contents, avoid these foods.

FOR GENERAL HYGIENE

- Wash your hands before and after handling any food.

- Thoroughly wash all fruit and vegetables, including ready-prepared salads, before eating. Peel and top carrots before eating them.

- Cook raw meat and poultry thoroughly and make sure that ready-to-eat poultry and cooked chilled meals are reheated thoroughly and are piping hot before they are eaten.

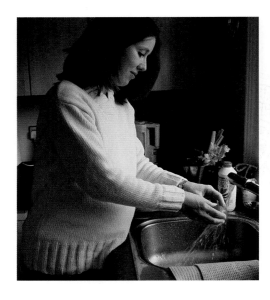

- Always wash your hands after handling raw meat or poultry and make sure that raw foods are stored separately from prepared foods. Otherwise there is a risk of contamination. Use a separate chopping board for raw meats.

- Wear gloves and wash them and then your hands thoroughly after gardening or handling soil.

- If you are in England or Wales ask your doctor or clinic for a copy of *Enjoy healthy eating*, a free booklet published by the Health Education Authority, and also the free Department of Health leaflet, *While you are pregnant: how to avoid infection from food and from contact with animals.* Other booklets may be available in Northern Ireland.

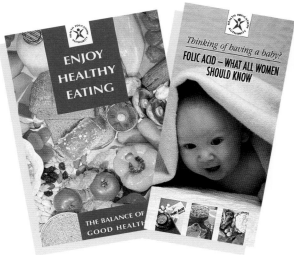

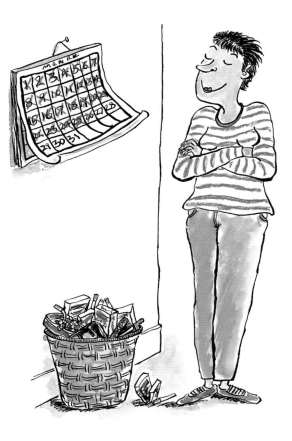

SMOKING

When you smoke, carbon monoxide and nicotine pass into your lungs and bloodstream. This means that: a) your baby gets less oxygen and cannot grow as well as it should, and b) the nicotine makes your baby's heart beat faster. Breathing in other people's smoke makes the baby more likely to suffer from asthma attacks, chest infections, coughs and colds, and to be admitted to hospital.

IF YOU STOP SMOKING NOW:

- you're more likely to have a healthier pregnancy and a healthier baby;

- you'll cope better with the birth;

- your baby will cope better with any birth complication;

- your baby is less likely to be born too early and have to face the additional breathing, feeding and health problems which so often go with prematurity (see page 112);

- your baby is less likely to be born underweight and have extra problems in keeping warm. Babies of mothers who smoke are, on average, 200 g (about 8 oz) lighter than other babies. These babies may have problems during and after labour and are more prone to infection;

- it will be better for your baby later too. Children whose parents smoke are more likely to suffer later on from illnesses which need hospital treatment (such as asthma);

- you will reduce the risk of cot death.

The sooner you stop, the better. But stopping even in the last few weeks of pregnancy can be beneficial. If any members of your household smoke, their smoke can affect you and the baby both before and after birth. They can help you and the baby by giving up now. Perhaps you could try to stop together.

Protecting the fetus and the new baby from tobacco smoke is one of the best things you can do to give your child a healthy start in life.

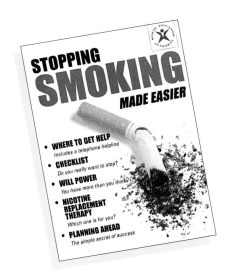

SMOKING
YOUR ACTION PLAN

Stop completely – it's never too late.

- **Choose a day.** *Will the first few days be easier during a working week or over a weekend? When you're busy or relaxed? Whatever you choose, stop completely on that day.*

- **The day before.** *Get everything ready; review your plan. Get rid of cigarettes.*

- **Get help.** *Ask friends for understanding and support. Consider asking your midwife, health visitor or practice nurse for advice.*

It might help to:

- *change the habits you associate with smoking;*

- *anticipate problems – plan to deal with difficult situations without the use of cigarettes;*

- *take one day at a time and reward yourself for success.*

You may need extra help: read the free Health Education Authority booklet, Stopping smoking made easier (other titles may be available in Northern Ireland), or phone Quitline on 0800 00 22 00; 0345 697500 in Wales, or the Ulster Cancer Foundation on 028 9066 3281 in Northern Ireland, for details of local support services.

ALCOHOL

There is no evidence that light or occasional drinking in pregnancy will harm your baby. But research shows that heavy or frequent drinking can seriously harm your baby's development. To be on the safe side, stop altogether or stick to no more than one or two 'units' of alcohol once or twice a week.

If you have difficulty cutting down, talk to your doctor or midwife. Confidential help and support is available from local counselling services (look in the telephone directory or contact Alcohol Concern). See page 143 for national agencies who can help.

1 UNIT EQUALS

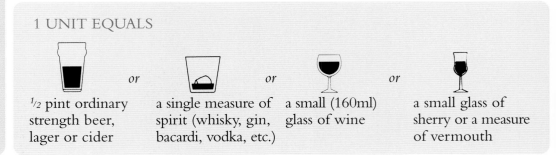

| ½ pint ordinary strength beer, lager or cider | *or* | a single measure of spirit (whisky, gin, bacardi, vodka, etc.) | *or* | a small (160ml) glass of wine | *or* | a small glass of sherry or a measure of vermouth |

These units apply to the 25 ml measure used in most of England and Wales. In some places, pub measures are larger than this. In Northern Ireland, a pub measure is 35 ml or 1½ units. In Scotland, it can either be 35 ml or 25 ml. Home measures are usually more generous.

PILLS, MEDICINES AND OTHER DRUGS

Some pills and medicines can harm your baby's health so, to be on the safe side, you should:

- assume that all medicines are dangerous until a doctor or pharmacist can tell you they are safe;

- make sure your doctor or dentist knows you're pregnant before prescribing anything or giving you treatment;

- talk to your doctor at the first possible moment if you take regular medication.

But do remember that it is safer to take some medicines, for example those used to treat epilepsy and diabetes, than to leave the illness untreated.

Illegal drugs (street drugs) can harm your baby. Taking cocaine or smoking crack may be especially harmful because both cause a sudden drop in blood and oxygen to the placenta. It's important to talk to your doctor or midwife straightaway so they can refer you to a maintenance reduction programme. For more information contact one of the organisations on page 143, or the National Drugs Helpline on 0800 776600.

X-rays should be avoided in pregnancy if possible. Make sure your dentist knows you are pregnant.

PHYSICAL ACTIVITY

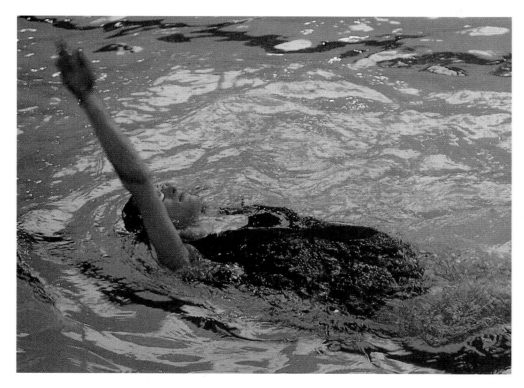

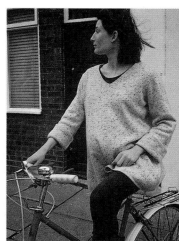

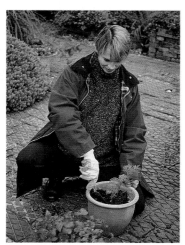

The more active and fit you are during pregnancy, the easier it will be for you to adapt to your changing shape and weight gain. It will also help you to cope with labour and get back into shape after the birth. If you feel tense after a hard day's work, physical activity is an excellent way of relaxing and it will help you to sleep soundly.

Keep up your normal daily physical activity or exercise (sport, or dancing, or just walking to the shops and back) for as long as you feel comfortable. Don't exhaust yourself and remember that you may need to slow down as your pregnancy progresses, or if your doctor advises you to. If in doubt, consult your doctor or midwife.

● If you were inactive before you were pregnant, don't suddenly take up strenuous exercise. Remember, exercise doesn't have to be strenuous to be beneficial.

● Try to keep active on a daily basis. Building in half an hour of activities like walking can help to keep you active. If you can't manage that, any amount is better than nothing.

● Avoid any strenuous exercise in hot weather.

● Drink plenty of fluids.

● If you go to exercise classes, make sure your teacher is properly qualified, and knows that you're pregnant and how far your pregnancy has progressed.

● You might like to try swimming because the water will support your increased weight. Some local swimming pools provide aquanatal classes with qualified instructors.

Every pregnant woman should try to fit these exercises into her daily routine. They will strengthen muscles to take a bigger load, make joints stronger, improve circulation, ease backache and generally make you feel well.

Stomach strengthening excercises
These strengthen abdominal muscles and eases backache, which can be a problem in pregnancy. As your baby gets bigger you may find that the hollow in your lower back increases. This can give you backache.

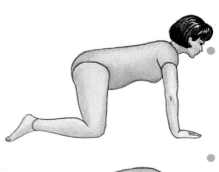

- Start in a box position (on all fours) with knees under hips, hands under shoulders with fingers facing forward and abdominals lifted to keep the back straight;

- pull in the abdominals and raise the back up towards the ceiling, curling the trunk and allowing the head to relax gently forward. Don't allow elbows to lock out;

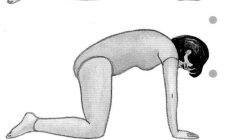

- hold for a few seconds then slowly return to the box position;

- take care not to hollow the back. The back should always return to a straight/neutral position;

- do this slowly and rhythmically ten times, making your muscles work hard and moving your back carefully. Only move your back as far as you can comfortably.

Pelvic floor exercises help strengthen the muscles of the pelvic floor which come under great strain in pregnancy and childbirth. The pelvic floor consists of layers of muscles which stretch like a supportive hammock from the pubic bone (in front) to the end of the backbone. If your pelvic floor muscles are weak, you may find that you leak urine when you cough or sneeze. This is quite common and you needn't feel embarrassed.

However, you can strengthen the muscles by doing the following exercise:

- close up your back passage as if trying to prevent a bowel movement;

- at the same time, draw in your vagina as if you are gripping a tampon, and your urethra as if to stop the flow of urine;

- hold for five seconds;

- repeat this exercise in sets of five, ten times a day.

Foot exercises can be done sitting or standing. They improve blood circulation, reduce swelling in the ankles, and prevent cramp in the calf muscles.

- Bend and stretch your foot vigorously up and down 30 times.

- Rotate your foot eight times one way and eight times the other way.

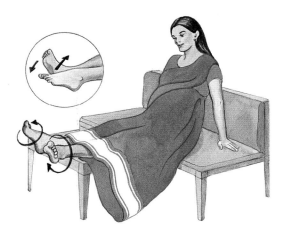

Protect your back

- Sit up straight with your bottom against the back of your chair. Tuck a small cushion behind your waist if you wish.

- When you pick something up, bend your knees, not your back.

- Try to stand tall.

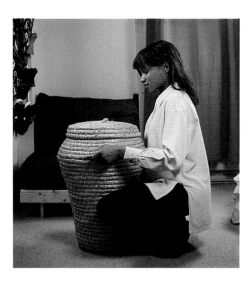

INFECTIONS

RUBELLA

Rubella (or German measles) can seriously affect your baby's sight and hearing and cause brain and heart defects in your baby if you catch it in the first four months of pregnancy. All children are now immunised against rubella at 12 to 15 months and again before they start school.

If you're not immune and you do come into contact with rubella, tell your doctor at once. Blood tests will show whether you have been infected, and you will then be better able to think about what action to take.

SEXUALLY TRANSMITTED INFECTIONS

Sexually transmitted infections (STIs) are very common and often there are no symptoms, so you may not know if you have one. However, many STIs can affect your baby's health during pregnancy and after birth. If you have any reason to believe that you or your partner could have an STI which was not diagnosed before pregnancy, you should go for a check-up as soon as you can. You can ask your GP or midwife or, if you prefer, go to a hospital clinic where you will also be guaranteed strict confidentiality. You can find your nearest clinic in your phone book, listed under the name of your health authority as genito-urinary medicine (GUM) clinic, or 'special' clinic, or the old name of venereal disease (VD) clinic.

REMEMBER THAT YOU CAN GET INFECTED BY HIV OR HEPATITIS B IF YOU:

- *have intercourse without using a condom, with anyone who is infected;*

- *use injectable drugs and share equipment with an infected person.*

HUMAN IMMUNO-DEFICIENCY VIRUS (HIV) AND ACQUIRED IMMUNE DEFICIENCY SYNDROME (AIDS)

Current evidence suggests that an HIV positive mother in good health and without symptoms of the infection is unlikely to be adversely affected by pregnancy. However, 15% of children born to HIV positive mothers are likely to be infected. HIV positive mothers may also pass on the virus through breast milk. If you're HIV positive, talk to your doctor about your own health and the options open to you, or contact the organisations listed on page 141 for advice and counselling. It is possible to reduce the risk of transmitting HIV to your baby during pregnancy and after birth (see page 54).

If you suspect that you or your partner could be at risk of HIV, ask your doctor, midwife or health visitor, or go to a special clinic (see above) for advice before you decide whether or not to have a blood test for HIV. If you have a test, counselling should be offered afterwards to explain the result and the implications if it is either positive or negative.

HEPATITIS B

Hepatitis B is an infection spread by contact with infected blood and body fluids, usually from sexual contact or from sharing needles. If you get hepatitis B when you are pregnant it can be passed on to the baby. Many hospitals screen for hepatitis B infection with a blood test. Babies who are at risk can be immunised at birth.

HERPES

Genital herpes infection can be dangerous for a newborn baby. It can be caught through genital contact with an infected person or from oral sex with someone who has oral herpes (cold sores). Initial infection causes very painful blisters, or ulcers on the genitals. Less severe recurrent attacks usually occur for some years afterwards. If you, or your partner, are infected, use condoms or avoid sex during an attack. Avoid oral sex if you or your partner have cold sores or active genital herpes. Tell your doctor or midwife if either you or your partner have recurring herpes or develop the symptoms described above. If your first infection occurs in pregnancy there is a treatment available, although its use is controversial. If the infection is active during labour, a Caesarean section may be recommended to reduce the risk of transmission to the baby.

CHICKEN POX

Around 95% of women are immune to chicken pox. If you have never had chicken pox, or are unsure, and come into contact with a child or adult who has it, speak to your GP, midwife or obstetrician at once. A blood test will establish if you are immune. Chicken pox infection in pregnancy can be dangerous for both mother and baby. so seek advice early.

TOXOPLASMOSIS

This infection can damage your baby if you catch it during pregnancy, so take precautions (see page 19). Most women have already had the infection before pregnancy and will be immune. If you feel you may have been at risk, discuss the matter with your GP, midwife or obstetrician. If you do catch toxoplasmosis while you are pregnant, treatment is available.

Parvovirus B19 (Slapped cheek disease)

Parvovirus B19 infection is common in children and causes a characteristic red rash on the face, so is often called 'slapped cheek disease'. Although 60% of women are immune to this infection, since parvovirus is highly infectious and can be harmful to the baby, any pregnant woman who comes into contact with someone who is infected should seek advice from the doctor. Immunity can be checked with a blood test. In most pregnant women who are infected with parvovirus the baby is not affected.

ANIMALS

Cats' faeces may contain an organism which causes **toxoplasmosis** – a disease which can damage your baby. Avoid emptying cat litter trays while you're pregnant or, if no one else can do it, use disposable rubber gloves. Trays should be cleaned daily and filled with boiling water for five minutes. Avoid close contact with sick cats and wear gloves when gardening –

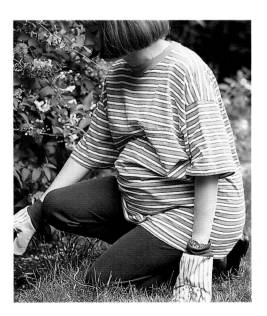

even if you don't have a cat – in case the soil is contaminated with faeces. Wash your hands and gloves after gardening. If you do come into contact with cat faeces, make sure you wash your hands thoroughly. Follow the general hygiene rules under **Take care with some foods** (page 11). For further information, contact the Toxoplasmosis Trust (see page 143).

Lambs and sheep can be a source of an organism called Chlamydia psittaci which is known to cause miscarriage in ewes. They also carry Toxoplasma. Avoid lambing or milking ewes and all contact with newborn lambs. If you experience flu-like symptoms after coming into contact with sheep, tell your doctor.

Ask your doctor or clinic for a copy of the leaflet, *While you are pregnant: how to avoid infection from food and from contact with animals.*

INHERITED CONDITIONS

Some diseases or conditions, like cystic fibrosis, haemophilia, muscular dystrophy, sickle cell disease and thalassaemia, are inherited from parents or grandparents. If you, your partner, or any relative has a condition which you know or suspect is inherited, or if you already have a baby with a disability, talk to your doctor about it. You may be able to have tests to check whether your baby is affected (see pages 52–4 and 55–7). Ask your GP to refer you to a genetic counsellor for specialist advice, if necessary, preferably before you conceive or in the early weeks of pregnancy.

WORK HAZARDS

VDUs

Some women are concerned about reports of the effects of VDUs (visual display units on computer terminals and word processors) in pregnancy. The most recent research shows no evidence of a risk.

If you work with chemicals, lead or X-rays, or in a job with a lot of lifting, you may be risking your health and the health of your baby. If you have any worries about this, you should talk to your doctor, midwife, occupational health nurse, your union representative or your personnel department.

If it is a known and recognised risk, it may be illegal for you to continue and your employer must offer you an alternative job, if one is available. If no job is available, your employer can dismiss you. However, this would not affect your rights to maternity pay and leave (see **Rights and benefits,** page 130).

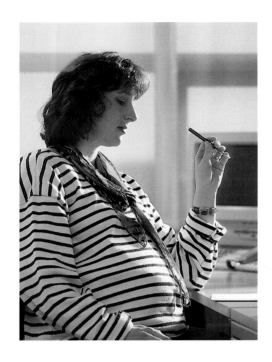

COPING AT WORK AND AT HOME

SAFETY ON THE MOVE

*Road accidents are among the most common causes of injury in pregnant women. To protect both you and your unborn baby, **always** wear a seatbelt with the diagonal strap across your body between your breasts and the lap belt over your upper thighs. The straps should lie above and below your 'bump', not over it.*

If you're at work during pregnancy you need to know your rights to antenatal care, leave and benefits which are set out on page 133–135. You may get extremely tired, particularly in the first and last weeks of your pregnancy. Try to use your lunch break to eat and rest, not to do the shopping. If travelling in rush hour is exhausting, ask your employer if you can work slightly different hours for a while.

Don't rush home and start another job cleaning and cooking. If possible, ask your partner to take over. If you're on your own, keep housework to a minimum, and go to bed early if you can.

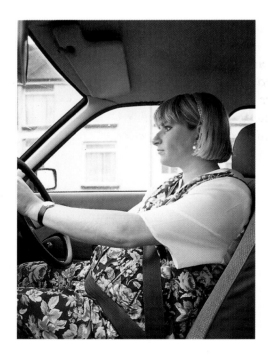

2 Conception

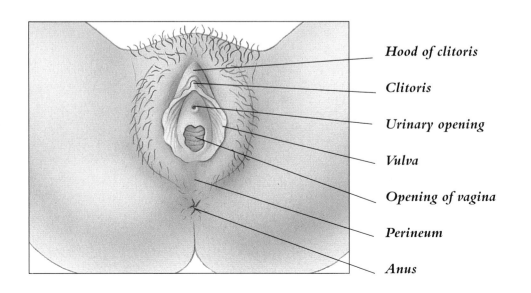

To understand about conception and pregnancy, it helps to know about the male and female sexual organs. This information is useful in pregnancy too, when you want to ask questions and be clear about what you are told.

THE MAN'S SEXUAL ORGANS

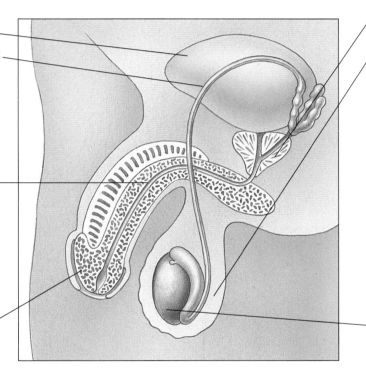

Bladder

Vas deferens *This tube carries sperm from the testes to the prostate and other glands. These glands add secretions which are ejaculated along with the sperm.*

Urethra *The urethra is a tube running down the length of the penis from the bladder, through the prostate gland to an opening at the tip of the penis. Sperm travel down the urethra to be ejaculated.*

Penis *The penis is made of erectile tissue. This tissue acts like a sponge and, when it becomes filled with blood, the penis becomes hard and erect.*

Prostate gland

Scrotum *This is the bag of skin which hangs outside the body and contains the testes. It helps to keep the testes at a constant temperature, just below the temperature of the rest of the body. This is necessary for sperm to be produced. In heat, the scrotum hangs down, away from the body, to keep the testes cool. When it is cold, the scrotum draws up closer to the body for warmth.*

Testes *There are two testes. These are where sperm are made.*

THE WOMAN'S SEXUAL ORGANS

Hood of clitoris

Clitoris

Urinary opening

Vulva

Opening of vagina

Perineum

Anus

21

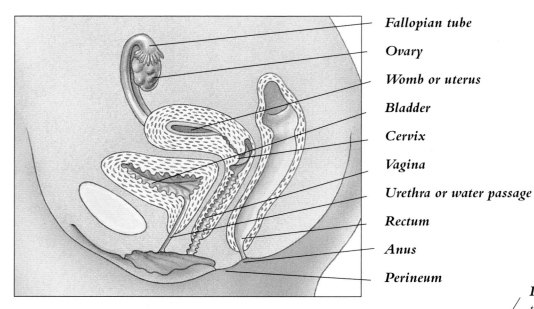

Fallopian tube

Ovary

Womb or uterus

Bladder

Cervix

Vagina

Urethra or water passage

Rectum

Anus

Perineum

Pelvis *The baby will pass through the pelvis when he or she is born.*

Womb or uterus *The womb is about the size and shape of a small upside down pear. It is made of muscle. It grows in size as the baby grows.*

Fallopian tubes *These lead from the ovaries to the womb.*

Ovaries *There are two ovaries, each about the size of an almond. They produce the eggs, or ova.*

Cervix *This is the neck of the womb. It is normally all but closed, with just a small opening through which blood passes during the monthly period.*

Vagina *The vagina is a tube about 8 cm (3 ins) long. It leads from the cervix down to the vulva, where it opens between the legs. The vagina is very elastic so it can easily stretch around a man's penis, or around a baby during labour.*

THE WOMAN'S MONTHLY CYCLE

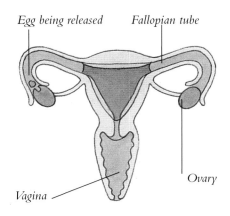

Egg being released   *Fallopian tube*

Vagina   *Ovary*

Egg progressing down the fallopian tube

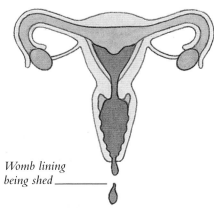

Womb lining being shed

1. *Each month a ripe egg or ovum (occasionally two) is released from one of the ovaries. This is called ovulation. The 'fingers' at the end of the fallopian tube help to direct the egg down into the tube. At the same time, the lining of the womb begins to thicken and the mucus in the cervix becomes thinner so that sperm can swim through it more easily.*

2. *The ripe egg begins to travel down the fallopian tube. It is here that it may be fertilised by a man's sperm if a couple have intercourse at this time. By now the lining of the womb is thick enough for the egg, if it is fertilised, to be implanted in it.*

3. *If the egg is not fertilised by a sperm, it passes out of the body through the vagina. It is so small that it cannot be seen. The lining of the womb is also shed in the monthly period of bleeding.*

CONCEPTION

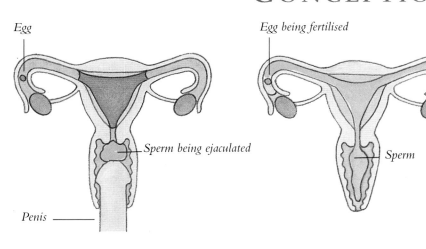

Egg

Sperm being ejaculated

Penis

Egg being fertilised

Sperm

Attached embryo

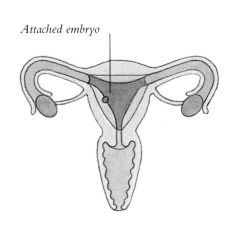

1. *A woman is most likely to conceive just after the time when she ovulates – when an egg has been released from one of her ovaries. During sexual intercourse, sperm are ejaculated from a man's penis into the woman's vagina. In one ejaculation, there may be more than 300 million sperm.*

2. *Most of the sperm leak out of the vagina again, but some begin to swim up through the cervix. At the time of ovulation the mucus in the cervix is thinner than usual to let the sperm pass through more easily. The sperm swim into the womb and so into the fallopian tube. One sperm may then join with the egg and fertilise it. Conception is said to have taken place.*

3. *During the week after fertilisation, the fertilised egg, or embryo, moves slowly down the fallopian tube and into the womb. It is already growing. The embryo attaches itself firmly to the specially thickened womb lining. Hormones released by the embryo and by the woman's ovary prevent shedding of the womb lining. The woman 'misses' her period.*

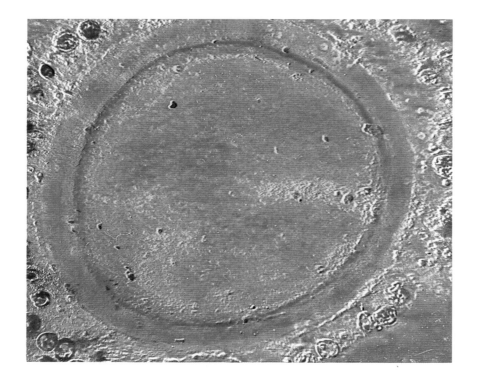

One ripe egg or ovum (occasionally two) is released from one of the woman's ovaries every month. It moves down into the fallopian tube where it may be fertilised by a man's sperm.

the events of the monthly cycle such as the release of the egg from the ovary and the thickening of the womb lining.

Once conception has occurred, the amount of oestrogen and progesterone increases. This causes the womb lining to build up, the blood supply to the womb and breasts to increase, and the muscles of the womb to relax to make room for the growing baby.

HORMONES

Hormones are chemicals which circulate in the blood of both men and women. They carry messages to different parts of the body, regulating certain activities and causing certain changes to take place. The female hormones, which include oestrogen and progesterone, control many of

A sperm is about 1/25th of a millimetre long and has a head, neck and tail. The tail moves from side to side so that the sperm can swim up the vagina into the womb and fallopian tubes.

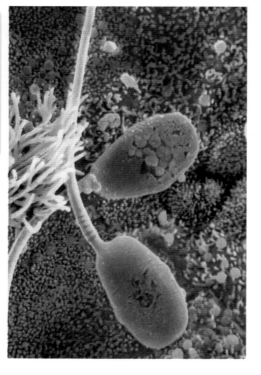

HEREDITY

Every normal human cell contains 46 chromosomes, except for the male sperm and female eggs. They contain 23 chromosomes each. When the sperm fuses with the egg and fertilisation takes place, the 23 chromosomes from the father pair with the 23 from the mother, making 46 in all.

The chromosomes are tiny thread-like structures which each carry about 2000 genes. It is the genes that determine the baby's inherited characteristics, such as hair and eye colour, blood group, height and build.

The fertilised egg contains one sex chromosome from the mother and one from the father. The sex chromosome from the mother's egg is always the same and is known as the X chromosome. But the sex chromosome from the father's sperm may be an X or a Y chromosome. If the egg is fertilised by a sperm containing an X chromosome, the baby will be a girl (XX). If the sperm contains a Y chromosome, then the baby will be a boy (XY).

THE BEST TIME TO GET PREGNANT

An egg lives for about 12 to 24 hours after it is released from the ovary. If conception is to take place it must be fertilised within this time. Sperm can live for several days inside the woman's body. If you make love a day or so before ovulation, the sperm will have time to travel up the fallopian tubes and will be waiting when the egg is released. So the chances are highest if you make love on the day before ovulation (see chart).

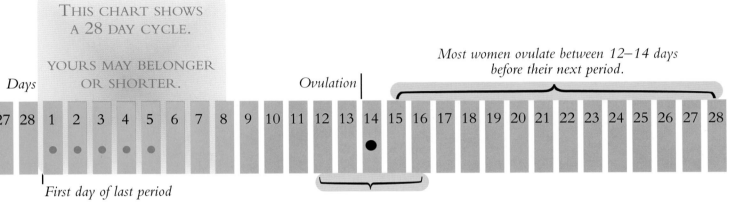

THIS CHART SHOWS
A 28 DAY CYCLE.

YOURS MAY BELONGER
OR SHORTER.

Days

Ovulation

Most women ovulate between 12–14 days before their next period.

| 27 | 28 | 1 | 2 | 3 | 4 | 5 | 6 | 7 | 8 | 9 | 10 | 11 | 12 | 13 | 14 | 15 | 16 | 17 | 18 | 19 | 20 | 21 | 22 | 23 | 24 | 25 | 26 | 27 | 28 |

First day of last period

You are most likely to conceive if you have intercourse about this time.

TWINS

Identical twins are the result of one fertilised egg splitting into two separate cells. Each cell grows into a baby. Because they originally came from the same cell, the babies have the same genes – they are the same sex and look very like each other. Non-identical twins are common. They are one result of two eggs being fertilised by two sperm at the same time. The babies may not be the same sex and will probably look no more alike than any other brothers and sisters.

Twins happen about once in every 80 pregnancies. A couple is more likely to have twins if there are twins in the woman's family. Triplets are much more rare and quads rarer still, although nowadays the use of drugs in the treatment of infertility has made multiple births more common. You may suspect that you are carrying twins if you are very sick in early pregnancy, seem bigger than your 'dates', they run in your family or you have had fertility treatment. It is usually possible to find out by about the end of the second month of your pregnancy. An ultrasound scan is needed (see page 56) to make the diagnosis at this stage. You should be told at this point whether the babies are in separate sacs or offered a further scan to determine this. Twin and other multiple pregnancies (e.g. triplets) carry a higher risk of most of the complications associated with pregnancy, particularly premature birth. You will probably be encouraged to have regular scans during your pregnancy to check the babies' growth. You may be advised to have a Caesarean section. Discuss this with your doctor. You can still breastfeed with twins. With triplets, or more, this may be more difficult.

It is a good idea to contact support groups like TAMBA (Twins and Multiple Births Association) and the Multiple Births Foundation (see pages 141 and 142) before the babies are born.

FINDING OUT IF YOU'RE PREGNANT

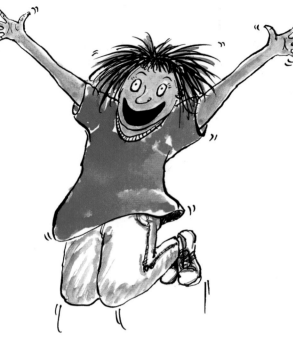

SEE YOUR DOCTOR

Whether or not you have had a pregnancy test, you should see your doctor as soon as you think you are pregnant. Being pregnant may affect your GP's treatment of any current or future illness. Your GP will also be able to advise you about antenatal care in your area and put you directly in touch with a midwife if you wish.

*Information about the services available is given in the chapters on **Deciding where to have your baby and Antenatal care and antenatal classes** (see pages 33 and 51). It may help to look at these chapters before you talk to your doctor.*

THE SIGNS OF PREGNANCY

The earliest and most reliable sign of pregnancy, for women who have a regular monthly cycle, is a missed period. Sometimes women who are pregnant have a very light period, losing only a little blood. Other signs of pregnancy are listed below.

- **Feeling sick** – you may feel sick, or even be sick, not necessarily in the morning, but at any time. If you are being sick all the time and can't keep anything down tell your doctor.

- **Changes in your breasts** – often the breasts become larger and feel tender, rather as they may do before a period. They may tingle. The veins may show up more and the nipples may darken and stand out.

- **Needing to pass water more often.** You may find that you have to get up in the night to do so.

- **Being constipated.**

  - An increased vaginal discharge without any soreness or irritation.

  - Feeling tired.

  - Having a strange taste in your mouth – many women describe it as metallic.

  - 'Going off' certain things like tea or coffee, tobacco smoke or fatty food, for example.

Some women don't even need these signs. They just 'know' that they are pregnant.

PREGNANCY TESTS

Pregnancy tests can be carried out on a sample of urine from the first day of a missed period – that is, about two weeks after conception. You can collect urine at any time of the day. Use a clean, soap-free, well-rinsed container to collect it. You can get pregnancy tests free or for a small charge from your GP or family planning clinic. Many pharmacists and most pregnancy advisory services also offer tests, usually for a small fee. You can also buy do-it-yourself pregnancy testing kits from pharmacists. They can be expensive but give you a quick result and you can do the test in private. Follow the instructions to be sure of a reliable result.

THE RESULTS OF THE TEST

A positive test result is almost certainly correct. A negative result is less reliable. You could wait a week

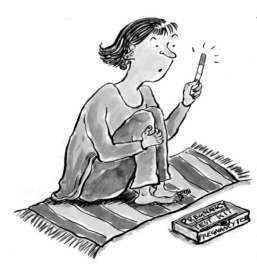

WORKING OUT WHEN YOUR BABY IS DUE

Use the chart below to work out your 'EDD' – expected date of delivery (or 'EDC' – expected date of confinement). Pick out the date of the first day of your last monthly period from the figures in black. The date your baby is due is immediately underneath it in blue.

For example, if your last period started on March 12, your baby will be due around December 17. Remember that this date is no more than a rough guide and it is based on a 28-day cycle. If your cycle is longer or shorter than this, your baby will be due later or earlier than the date shown in blue. In fact only 3% of babies are born on their 'due' date. 90% deliver in the week before or after the EDD.

January	1	2	3	4	5	6	7	8	9	10	11	12	13	14	15	16	17	18	19	20	21	22	23	24	25	26	27	28	29	30	31	January
October	8	9	10	11	12	13	14	15	16	17	18	19	20	21	22	23	24	25	26	27	28	29	30	31	1	2	3	4	5	6	7	November
February	1	2	3	4	5	6	7	8	9	10	11	12	13	14	15	16	17	18	19	20	21	22	23	24	25	26	27	28				February
November	8	9	10	11	12	13	14	15	16	17	18	19	20	21	22	23	24	25	26	27	28	29	30	1	2	3	4	5				December
March	1	2	3	4	5	6	7	8	9	10	11	12	13	14	15	16	17	18	19	20	21	22	23	24	25	26	27	28	29	30	31	March
December	6	7	8	9	10	11	12	13	14	15	16	17	18	19	20	21	22	23	24	25	26	27	28	29	30	31	1	2	3	4	5	January
April	1	2	3	4	5	6	7	8	9	10	11	12	13	14	15	16	17	18	19	20	21	22	23	24	25	26	27	28	29	30		April
January	6	7	8	9	10	11	12	13	14	15	16	17	18	19	20	21	22	23	24	25	26	27	28	29	30	31	1	2	3	4		February
May	1	2	3	4	5	6	7	8	9	10	11	12	13	14	15	16	17	18	19	20	21	22	23	24	25	26	27	28	29	30	31	May
February	5	6	7	8	9	10	11	12	13	14	15	16	17	18	19	20	21	22	23	24	25	26	27	28	1	2	3	4	5	6	7	March
June	1	2	3	4	5	6	7	8	9	10	11	12	13	14	15	16	17	18	19	20	21	22	23	24	25	26	27	28	29	30		June
March	8	9	10	11	12	13	14	15	16	17	18	19	20	21	22	23	24	25	26	27	28	29	30	31	1	2	3	4	5	6		April
July	1	2	3	4	5	6	7	8	9	10	11	12	13	14	15	16	17	18	19	20	21	22	23	24	25	26	27	28	29	30	31	July
April	8	9	10	11	12	13	14	15	16	17	18	19	20	21	22	23	24	25	26	27	28	29	30	31	1	2	3	4	5	6	7	May
August	1	2	3	4	5	6	7	8	9	10	11	12	13	14	15	16	17	18	19	20	21	22	23	24	25	26	27	28	29	30	31	August
May	8	9	10	11	12	13	14	15	16	17	18	19	20	21	22	23	24	25	26	27	28	29	30	31	1	2	3	4	5	6	7	June
September	1	2	3	4	5	6	7	8	9	10	11	12	13	14	15	16	17	18	19	20	21	22	23	24	25	26	27	28	29	30		September
June	8	9	10	11	12	13	14	15	16	17	18	19	20	21	22	23	24	25	26	27	28	29	30	1	2	3	4	5	6	7		July
October	1	2	3	4	5	6	7	8	9	10	11	12	13	14	15	16	17	18	19	20	21	22	23	24	25	26	27	28	29	30	31	October
July	8	9	10	11	12	13	14	15	16	17	18	19	20	21	22	23	24	25	26	27	28	29	30	31	1	2	3	4	5	6	7	August
November	1	2	3	4	5	6	7	8	9	10	11	12	13	14	15	16	17	18	19	20	21	22	23	24	25	26	27	28	29	30		November
August	8	9	10	11	12	13	14	15	16	17	18	19	20	21	22	23	24	25	26	27	28	29	30	31	1	2	3	4	5	6		September
December	1	2	3	4	5	6	7	8	9	10	11	12	13	14	15	16	17	18	19	20	21	22	23	24	25	26	27	28	29	30	31	December
September	8	9	10	11	12	13	14	15	16	17	18	19	20	21	22	23	24	25	26	27	28	29	30	31	1	2	3	4	5	6	7	October

KNOWING THAT YOU'RE PREGNANT

You may feel very happy or excited when you discover that you are pregnant, but you shouldn't worry if you don't. Even if you have been looking forward to pregnancy, it is not unusual for your feelings to take you by surprise. And if your pregnancy was unplanned, then you may feel quite confused. Give yourself a little time to adjust to the idea of being pregnant. Even though you may feel rather anxious and uncertain now, this does not mean that you won't come to enjoy your pregnancy or to welcome the idea of the baby. Discuss your feelings with your midwife or doctor who will help you to adjust to your pregnancy, or, in England and Wales, will give you advice if you are not happy to continue with it. You may want to share the news with family and friends immediately or wait a while until you've sorted out how you feel. Others in your family/extended family may have mixed feelings. You'll need to talk about these feelings. But do begin to think about your antenatal care (that is, the care you'll receive leading up to the birth of your baby) and where you would like to have your baby. The earlier you begin to organise this, the more chance you will have of getting what you want.

'I thought when I first got pregnant, "This is fantastic, it's really different, it's never happened to me before." '

'I wasn't very pleased at first. I was a bit shocked, I think, more than anything, and it took me about three months to get used to the idea that I was pregnant. I don't think I could believe it at first.'

27

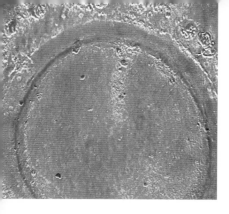

3 How the baby develops

Doctors and midwives in the UK time pregnancy from the first day of a woman's last menstrual period, not from conception. So what is called 'four weeks' pregnant' is actually about two weeks after conception. Pregnancy normally lasts for 37 to 42 weeks from the first day of your last period. The average is 40 weeks. If you're not sure about the date of your last period, then an ultrasound scan (see page 56) may give a good indication of when your baby will be due.

Week 1

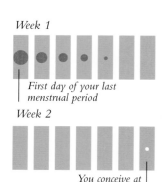

First day of your last menstrual period

Week 2

You conceive at about this time

Week 3

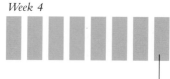

Week 4

At this point you will be called 4 weeks' pregnant

HOW THE BABY DEVELOPS

In the very early weeks, the developing baby is called an embryo. Then, from about eight weeks onward, it is called a fetus, meaning 'young one'.

Fertilised egg dividing and travelling down fallopian tube

WEEK 3

(Three weeks from the first day of your last menstrual period.) The fertilised egg moves slowly along the fallopian tube towards the womb. The egg begins as one single cell. This cell divides again and again. By the time the egg reaches the womb it has become a mass of over 100 cells, called an embryo, and is still growing. Once in the womb, the embryo burrows into the womb lining. This is called implantation.

Egg being fertilised

Egg being released from ovary

Ovary

Embryo implanting in womb lining

WEEKS 4–5

Week 4
ACTUAL SIZE ABOUT 5 MM

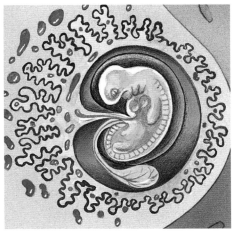

The embryo now settles into the womb lining. The outer cells reach out like roots to link with the mother's blood supply. The inner cells form into two and then later into three layers. Each of these layers will grow to be different parts of the baby's body. One layer becomes the brain and nervous system, the skin, eyes and ears. Another layer becomes the lungs, stomach and gut. The third layer becomes the heart, blood, muscles and bones.

The fifth week is the time of the first missed period when most women are only just beginning to think they may be pregnant. Yet already the baby's nervous system is starting to develop. A groove forms in the top layer of cells. The cells fold up and round to make a hollow tube called the neural tube. This will become the baby's brain and spinal cord, so the tube has a 'head end' and a 'tail end'. Defects in this tube are the cause of spina bifida.

At the same time the heart is forming and the baby already has some of its own blood vessels. A string of these blood vessels connects baby and mother and will become the umbilical cord.

WEEKS 6–7

There is now a large bulge where the heart is and a bump for the head because the brain is developing. The heart begins to beat and can be seen beating on an ultrasound scan.

Dimples on the side of the head will become the ears and there are thickenings where the eyes will be. On the body, bumps are forming which will become muscles and bones. And small swellings (called 'limb buds') show where the arms and legs are growing.

At seven weeks the embryo has grown to about 10 mm long from head to bottom. (This measurement is called the 'crown–rump length'.)

Week 6
ACTUAL SIZE HEAD TO BOTTOM ABOUT 8 MM

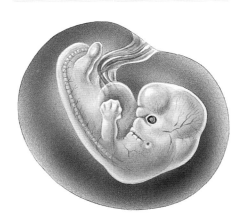

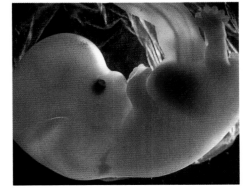

Week 7
ACTUAL SIZE HEAD TO BOTTOM ABOUT 10 MM

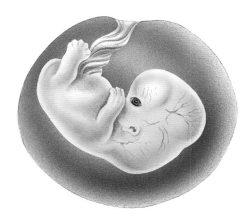

WEEKS 8–9

A face is slowly forming. The eyes are more obvious and have some colour in them. There is a mouth, with a tongue.

There are now the beginnings of hands and feet, with ridges where the fingers and toes will be.

The major internal organs are all devloping – the heart, brain, lungs, kidneys, liver and gut.

At nine weeks, the baby has grown to about 22 mm long from head to bottom.

Week 9
ACTUAL SIZE HEAD TO BOTTOM ABOUT 22 MM

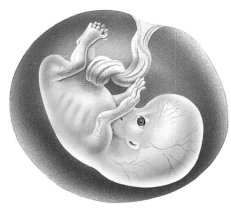

29

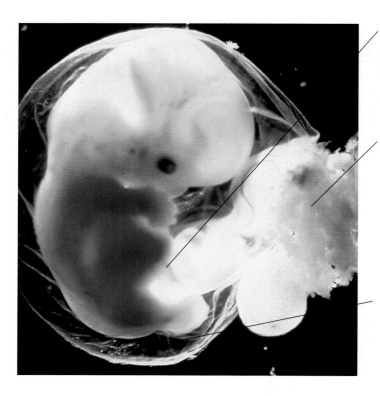

The umbilical cord

The umbilical cord is the baby's lifeline, the link between baby and mother. Blood circulates through the cord, carrying oxygen and food to the baby and carrying waste away again.

The placenta

The placenta is rooted to the lining of the womb and separates the baby's circulation from the mother's. In the placenta, oxygen and food from the mother's bloodstream pass across into the baby's bloodstream and are carried to the baby along the umbilical cord. Antibodies, giving resistance to infection, pass to the baby in the same way, but so too can alcohol, nicotine and other drugs.

The amniotic sac

Inside the womb the baby floats in a bag of fluid called the amniotic sac. Before or during labour the sac, or 'membranes', break and the fluid drains out. This is called the 'waters breaking'.

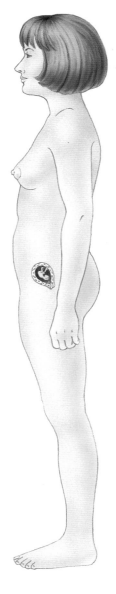

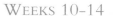

> **Week 14**
> ACTUAL SIZE HEAD TO BOTTOM ABOUT 85 MM

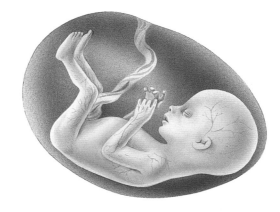

WEEKS 10–14

Just 12 weeks after conception the fetus is fully formed. It has all its organs, muscles, limbs and bones, and its sex organs are well developed. From now on it has to grow and mature.

The baby is already moving about, but the movements cannot yet be felt.

By about 14 weeks, the heartbeat is strong and can be heard using an ultrasound detector. The heartbeat is very fast – about twice as fast as a normal adult's heartbeat.

At 14 weeks the baby is about 85 mm long from head to bottom. The pregnancy may be just beginning to show, but this varies a lot from woman to woman.

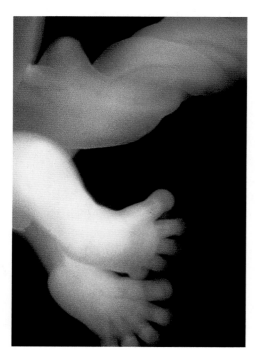

WEEKS 15-22

The baby is now growing quickly. The body grows bigger so that the head and body are more in proportion and the baby doesn't look so top heavy. The face begins to look much more human and the hair is beginning to grow as well as eyebrows and eyelashes. The eyelids stay closed over the eyes.

The lines on the skin of the fingers are now formed, so the baby already has its own individual fingerprint. Finger and toenails are growing and the baby has a firm hand grip.

At about 22 weeks, the baby becomes covered in a very fine, soft hair called 'lanugo'. The purpose of this isn't known, but it is thought that it may be to keep the baby at the right temperature. The lanugo disappears before birth, though sometimes just a little is left and disappears later.

At about 16 to 22 weeks you will feel your baby move for the first time. If this is your second baby, you may feel it earlier – at about 16 to 18 weeks after conception. At first you feel a fluttering or bubbling, or a very slight shifting movement, maybe a bit like indigestion. Later you can't mistake the movements and you can even see the baby kicking about. Often you can guess which bump is a hand or a foot and so on.

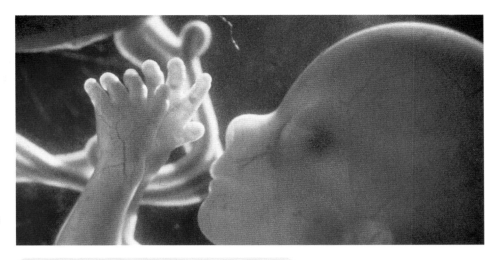

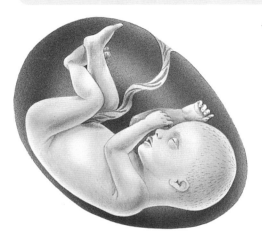

Week 22
ACTUAL SIZE HEAD TO BOTTOM ABOUT 27 CM

WEEKS 23–30

The baby is now moving about vigorously and responds to touch and to sound. A very loud noise close by may make it jump and kick. It is also swallowing small amounts of the amniotic fluid in which it is floating and passing tiny amounts of urine back into the fluid. Sometimes the baby may get hiccups and you can feel the jerk of each hiccup. The baby may also begin to follow a pattern for waking and sleeping. Very often this is a different pattern from yours so, when you go to bed at night, the baby wakes up and starts kicking.

The baby's heartbeat can now be heard through a stethoscope. Your partner may even be able to hear it by putting an ear to your abdomen,

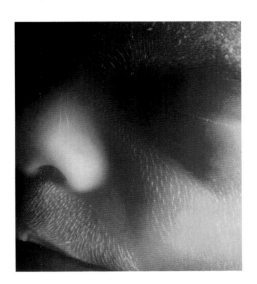

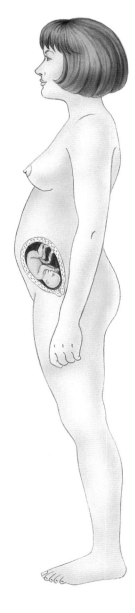

31

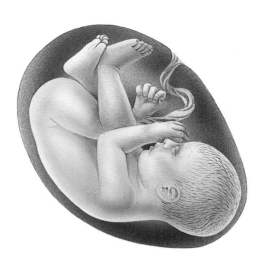

Week 30
ACTUAL SIZE HEAD
TO BOTTOM ABOUT 33 CM

but it can be difficult to find the right place. The baby is now covered in a white, greasy substance called 'vernix'. It is thought that this may be to protect the baby's skin as it floats in the amniotic fluid. The vernix mostly disappears before the birth.

At 24 weeks, the baby is called 'viable'. This means that the baby is now thought to have a chance of survival if born. Most babies born before this time cannot live because their lungs and other vital organs are not well enough developed. The care that can now be given in neonatal units means that more and more babies born early do survive.

At around 26 weeks the baby's eyelids open for the first time. The eyes are almost always blue or dark blue. It is not until some weeks after birth that the eyes become the colour they will stay, although some babies do have brown eyes at birth. The head to bottom length at 30 weeks is about 33 cm.

WEEKS 31–40

The baby is growing plumper so the skin, which was quite wrinkled before, is now smoother. Both the vernix and the lanugo begin to disappear.

By about 32 weeks the baby is usually lying downwards ready for birth. Some time before birth, the head may move down into the pelvis and is said to be 'engaged', but sometimes the baby's head does not engage until labour has started.

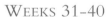

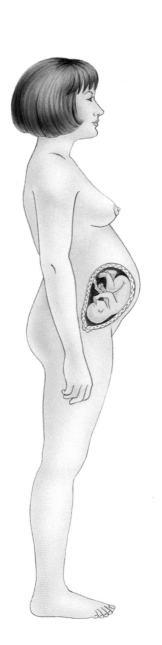

4 Deciding where to have your baby

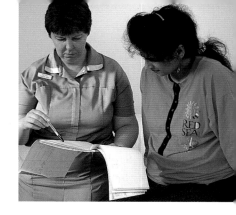

T he choice you have about where to have your baby and how you are cared for will depend to some extent on where you live. But what should be the same everywhere is that the care and the place should feel right for you.

It's important for you to make **informed** choices about the sort of care you would like and where you would like to give birth. Try to get information from as many sources as possible. You can go and look round the local hospital where there will probably be information leaflets about the services on offer. Midwives and your GP's surgery should also be able to tell you about the different options for care available in your area.

Don't hesitate to ask questions if you don't understand something or if you think that you need to know more. Midwives and doctors are there to help and support you. They want to make you feel as comfortable as possible with all aspects of the care you receive, both while you are pregnant and when you have your baby.

When you find out (or think) that you are pregnant, you can go either to your GP or direct to a midwife to discuss and arrange your care. Once you have found out what's available locally, talk things over with your GP or midwife. They will be able to offer you advice based on your

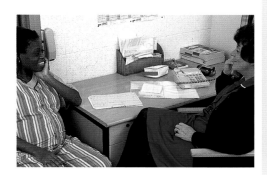

medical history and any previous pregnancies you may have had but, remember, the choice is yours. Don't forget, if you make your choice and then think that some other sort of care would be better for you and your baby, you can change your mind.

Your basic options will be to have your baby:

- in a **hospital** (a specialist unit with consultant obstetricians);

- at **home**;

- in a **GP/midwife unit** (either as part of a large general hospital, in a smaller community hospital, or completely separate).

SEE YOUR MIDWIFE OR DOCTOR AS SOON AS POSSIBLE IF:

- *you are currently being treated for a chronic disease, such as diabetes or epilepsy;*

- *you are over 35, so that you can be offered additional tests for abnormalities in the baby;*

- *you are a teenager – there may be services available to you specifically for your age group;*

- *you have previously had a baby with spina bifida, Down's syndrome, or you have a family history of a genetic disorder such as cystic fibrosis or sickle cell disease – additional tests will be offered to you;*

- *you have previously had an ectopic pregnancy – you may be able to have an ultrasound scan to check that the pregnancy is in the womb.*

33

THE BASIC OPTIONS

HOW TO BOOK IN FOR A HOSPITAL DELIVERY

Your GP or midwife will either send a letter to the hospital or give you one to take there. This is best done as early in your pregnancy as possible.

Ask your GP or midwife for the Department of Health's leaflet, How to get the best from maternity services. (This is not available in Northern Ireland.)

Spend some time thinking about the following options. Discuss them before you come to a decision.

IN HOSPITAL

For the last 30 years most babies have been born in hospital. Many hospitals have tried hard to meet parents' wishes and to make labour and delivery as private and special as possible. All over the country maternity care staff are working even harder to make sure that women get kind, sympathetic and sensitive care. Hospital maternity units should become friendlier, more comfortable places, where you will be able to get to know the people who are caring for you. You will probably be asked many questions about your wishes so you should feel more in control over what's happening to you.

If there is more than one hospital in your district, and you can choose which to go to, try to find out about the practice in each so that you can decide which will suit you best. **Team midwifery** may be in operation which means that you will see a midwife from the same team each time you visit the hospital, including at the delivery of your baby. Or there may be a **Domino Scheme** which means that your midwife will attend you at home in labour, accompany you to hospital to deliver your baby, and then accompany you home after the delivery (usually six hours later). Midwifery care will then continue to be provided as necessary for 10 to 28 days.

Use the checklist on page 36 as a guide to the sort of questions to ask. Talk to your doctor or midwife. It's also a good idea to talk to other mothers who have recently had babies and ask them about their

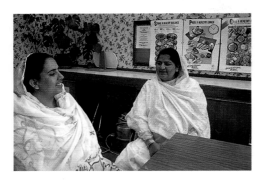

experiences at local hospitals. You can contact other mothers through your local branch of the National Childbirth Trust, your local Community Health Council and AIMS (the Association for Improvements in the Maternity Services), see page 141.

AT HOME

Some women want to have their babies at home because:

- they feel they will be happier and better able to cope in a place they know and with their family around them;

- if they have other young children, there will be no need to leave them to go into hospital;

- they will have more privacy;

- they will be able to relax more and will not have to fit into a hospital routine;

- they are more likely to get to know the midwife who will be with them during the delivery.

One or two midwives will stay with you while you're in labour and, if any help is needed or labour is not progressing as well as it should, will summon a doctor or transfer you to hospital by ambulance.

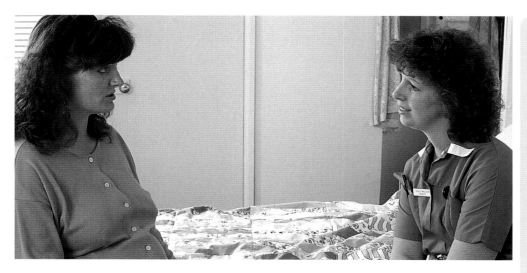

How to arrange for a home delivery

If you are considering a home delivery, first talk to your midwife and GP. Some people think that women should not have home births because they argue that they are unsafe. In fact, research suggests that a home delivery is as safe as a hospital delivery for women who have uncomplicated pregnancies. You have the right to choose to have your baby at home. Your doctor or midwife may advise against this if they think that you are at risk of complications during labour. However, this may be difficult to judge if this is your first baby.

Find out whether your own GP will be prepared to care for you during your pregnancy and a home delivery. If he or she cannot help, there may be another in the district who can. You can then register with this GP just for your maternity care and continue to see your own GP for any other medical treatment. The local supervisor of midwives (see box) or Local Health Authority can give you the names of GPs with a special interest in pregnancy and childbirth.

Alternatively, it is possible to arrange for maternity care to be led by a team of midwives. Contact the local supervisor of midwives at your nearest hospital who will arrange for a midwife to visit you at home to discuss home delivery. The midwife may also be able to provide most or all of your antenatal care at home. You can contact her directly when labour starts and she will stay with you during labour and the birth of your baby.

In a GP or midwife unit

This may be part of the hospital's ordinary maternity wards or a separate unit. Your baby can be delivered here by your community midwife, who has been involved in your antenatal care, and your GP (or sometimes by a hospital midwife). Some areas operate a **team midwifery** system (see page 34), so you may get to know who will deliver your baby.

Care in a GP or midwife unit can be more personal since you will usually be looked after by people you know. If the unit is part of the main hospital, then emergency facilities are there, should an unforeseen problem arise. This type of unit is generally used for women who are likely to have a normal delivery. The length of time you will remain in the unit after the birth depends on how well you and your baby are.

YOU CAN ALSO ASK FOR INFORMATION ON YOUR OPTIONS FROM:

- *any other* **health professional**, *particularly your midwife or health visitor – your GP or the Child Health Clinic can put you in touch with them;*

- *the* **local supervisor of midwives,** *who is also usually a senior midwife at the local maternity or district general hospital – you can get in touch through your health authority or hospital and the addresses and telephone numbers will be in your local phone book;*

- *your local* **Community Health Council** *(see page 141); in Northern Ireland your local Health and Social Services Council;*

- *your local branch of the* **National Childbirth Trust** *(see page 141);*

- *the* **Association for Improvements in the Maternity Services** *(AIMS) (see page 141);*

- **friends.**

35

*Before you try to get answers to your questions and make your decision, it will help to read the chapter on **Labour and birth** (page 89).*

THESE ARE THE KINDS OF QUESTIONS YOU MAY WISH TO ASK ABOUT A HOSPITAL

Would I go to the hospital antenatal clinic for all or just some of my antenatal care appointments?

Does the antenatal clinic run an appointments system?

Does the hospital run antenatal classes?

Does the hospital offer team midwifery care or the Domino Scheme for delivery (see page 34)?

Will I be shown round the labour and postnatal wards before the birth?

Is there a chance for me to discuss and work out a birth plan?

Can I be seen by a woman doctor if I prefer?

ABOUT LABOUR AND DELIVERY

Are fathers, close relatives or friends welcome in the delivery room?

Are they ever asked to leave the room, and why?

Does the hospital encourage women to move around in labour and find their own position for the birth, if that is what they want?

What is the hospital policy on induction, pain relief, routine monitoring, diet or any other aspect of labour that concerns me?

AFTERWARDS

Are babies usually put to their mother's breast immediately after birth?

What services are provided for sick babies?

Are babies with their mothers all the time or is there a separate nursery?

Will the hospital encourage (and help) me to feed my baby 'on demand' if this is what I want to do?

Who will help me breastfeed my baby?

Will I get help if I choose to bottle feed?

What is the normal length of stay?

What are visiting hours?

Are there any special rules about visiting?

Birth plan

A birth plan is a record of what you would like to happen during your labour and after the birth. You may be given an opportunity to draw up a birth plan during your antenatal care. If not, ask your midwife if you can do so. Discussing a birth plan with your midwife, preferably over several meetings, will give you the chance to ask questions and find out more information. It also gives the midwife the chance to get to know you better and understand your feelings and priorities. You will probably want to think about or discuss some points more fully with your partner, or friends and relatives, before reaching a decision. And you can, of course, change your mind at any time.

There is no one, correct way to give birth. All birth plans have to be drawn up individually and then discussed with your midwife. They depend not only on your own wishes, but also on your medical history and your own circumstances, and on what is available at your own hospital or unit. What may be safe and practical for one mother may not be a good idea for another.

You may be given a special form for a birth plan, or there may be room in your notes. You could use page 38 of this book as a guide. It's a good idea for you to keep a copy of your birth plan with you. The midwife or doctor who cares for you during labour will discuss it with you so they know your wishes. But remember, you may need to be flexible if complications arise with you or the baby. The doctor or midwife will tell you what they advise in your particular circumstances. Don't hesitate to ask questions if you need to.

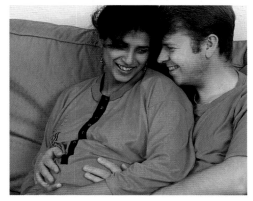

Read the chapters on **Labour and birth** (page 89) and **The first days with your new baby** (page 107) before talking to your midwife, to see if there is anything you feel strongly about and might wish to include. You may find it useful to think about some of these things. You may want to take this book with you to discuss with your midwife.

BREASTFEEDING

If you have decided to breastfeed, your birth plan should note that you want to put your baby to your breast straight after birth. This helps to get breastfeeding started. It should also note that you do not want your baby to be given any extra formula milk feeds, as this can hinder successful breastfeeding.

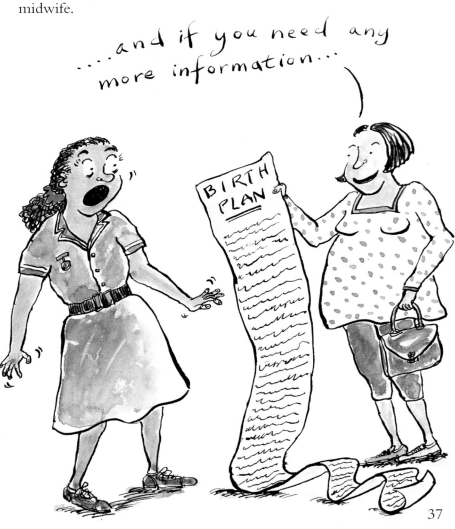

37

BIRTH PLAN

Do you want your partner, or a chosen companion(s), to be with you during labour?

Do you want your partner or companion to be with you if you have a Caesarean section or forceps delivery, for example?

Is equipment such as mats, a birthing chair or beanbags available to you if you want it, or can you bring your own?

Are there special facilities, like special rooms or birthing pools?

How do you want your baby's heart monitored if everything is straightforward?

Do you prefer to be cared for and delivered by women only?

Is it important for you to be able to move around when you're in labour?

What position would you like to be in for the birth?

If you think you would like pain relief, which sort do you want to try (see page 91)? If you want to try to manage without pain relief, it's a good idea to note this in the birth plan too.

Are epidurals available at all times should you want one?

Are there other means, such as warm baths, massage or other therapies, that you would like to use to help you cope with labour?

What do you feel about an episiotomy?

Do you want your baby delivered straight on to your tummy or do you want your baby cleaned first?

Do you have any feelings about the injection Syntocinon or Syntometrine usually given to you after the birth to help the womb contract?

How do you wish to feed your baby?

Do you want your baby close to you all the time? If you intend to breastfeed you should make a note that you want your baby close by you all the time or brought to you when hungry so that you can feed on demand.

Do you want your baby to have vitamin K, and by which route (see page 110)?

Is there anything you feel you may need extra help with?

Do you mind if students are present?

Do you need an interpreter?

Do you need a sign language interpreter?

Do you need a special diet?

Do you or your partner or companion have special needs that should be considered, for example, do you or your partner normally use a guide dog or a wheelchair?

Are there special religious customs you wish to be observed?

5 Feelings and relationships

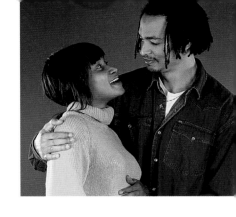

From the minute you know you're pregnant, things begin to change. Your feelings change – feelings about yourself, about the baby, about your future. Your relationships change – with your partner, other children and also with parents and friends.

But you're still yourself, and you still have to get on with your life, whether pregnant or not. For this reason, adjusting to the changes that pregnancy brings isn't always easy. This chapter is about some of the worries that may crop up in pregnancy and some suggestions on how to handle them. But, of course, what may be a problem for one person may not be a problem for another. And what is helpful advice for some people may not be right for you. So take from these pages what you find useful, and don't bother about the rest.

'I think you have more extremes of emotion. You get more easily upset about things, and you can more easily get very happy about things.'

FEELINGS

When you're pregnant it can sometimes seem as though you are not allowed to have other feelings as well. People expect you to be looking forward to the baby, to be excited and to 'bloom' all the time. You, yourself, may think that this is the way you ought to be. In fact, just like any other nine months in your life, you're likely to have times when you feel low. And pregnancy does bring extra reasons for feeling worried or down,

just as it brings many reasons for happiness.

'It frightens me, wondering what I've got to go through. People say different things, you know, so you don't know what to think.'

'I think it's a lot to do with mind over matter. I think the thing to do is just try and relax and not be frightened. I mean, it's happened to thousands and millions of people before you.'

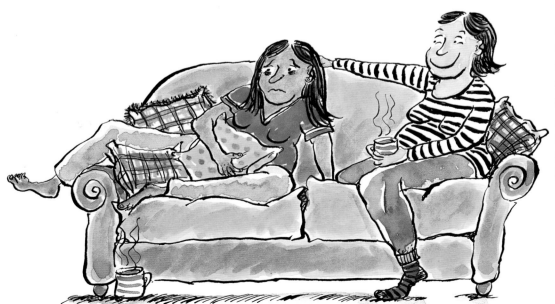

'I've enjoyed it. I've enjoyed the newness of it. I've enjoyed thinking of the baby. The only thing I haven't enjoyed is getting so big.'

'I loved every minute of being pregnant and went through a wonderful experience with labour.'

'Antenatal classes really helped. I met lots of women there who had the same fears as me. The midwife made us more confident by telling us what happens in labour. I felt well prepared.'

Hormonal changes taking place in your body are responsible for much of the tiredness and nausea that some women feel in the early months and for some of the emotional upsets which can happen. You may find you cry more easily, lose your temper more, and so on.

Of course, there are many other reasons why you may feel rather down. You may have money worries or worries about work or where you are going to live. You may be anxious about whether you will cope as a parent, or about whether you're really ready to be a parent at all. And many of these anxieties may be shared by your partner or family as well. This may be your first baby but not your partner's so you may see and feel things differently. Talk through these feelings together.

Talking about your feelings to your partner, or to someone who is close to you, is often a relief and can help you get things in proportion. It may help your partner too. Making sure you keep yourself well and get plenty of sleep will also help. Anyone who is tired

WORRYING ABOUT THE BIRTH

One worry that a lot of women have in pregnancy is whether labour and birth will be painful and how they will cope. It is difficult to imagine what a contraction might be like and no one can tell you – though many will try. However, factual information about the options open to you can help you to feel more confident and more in control.

Begin by reading the chapter on **Labour and birth** (page 89) with your partner, or a friend or relative who will be with you for the birth, if possible. Ask your midwife or doctor for any further information. Antenatal classes will also help to prepare you for labour and the birth (see pages 64–5).

Think about the sort of labour and birth you would like to have. You will probably have an opportunity to discuss this in more detail with your midwife and to draw up a birth plan during the later months of pregnancy (see page 38).

Talk to your partner too, or to someone close to you, and particularly to the person who will

be with you in labour. Remember they may be anxious also. Together you can then work out ways in which to cope.

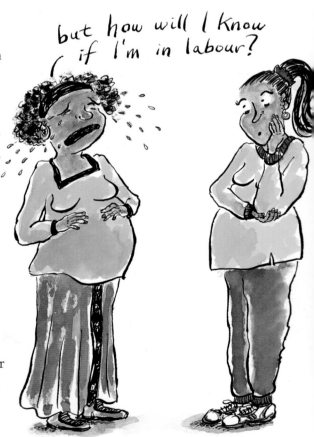

but how will I know if I'm in labour?

WORRYING ABOUT ABNORMALITY

Everyone worries at some time that there may be something wrong with their baby. Some people find that talking openly about their fears helps them to cope. Others prefer not to dwell on the possibility of something being wrong.

Some women continue to worry because they are convinced that if something does go wrong it will be their fault. While you can increase your baby's chances of being born healthy by following the advice outlined in Chapter 1 (see pages 8–20), you cannot cut out the risk entirely. There are certain problems which cannot be prevented, either because the causes are not known or because they are beyond anyone's control.

It may reassure you to know that 97% of babies born in the UK are normal, although some of these may have birthmarks or some other small variations. A further 1% of babies will be born with abnormalities that can be partly or completely corrected. About 2%, however, will suffer from some more severe disability. Regular antenatal care and careful observation during labour help so that action can be taken if necessary.

If you are particularly concerned, perhaps because someone in your family has a disability, or because someone you know has had a difficult birth, or even if you just feel very anxious, talk to your doctor or midwife as soon as possible. They may be able to reassure you or offer you helpful information about tests which can be done in pregnancy (see pages 53–9).

'I want to know if it's all right. I think that's always at the back of your mind – you don't know whether it's all right. It's a worry that's always there.'

'I feel guilty at times. It's not just worrying about what you do and whether it will damage the baby. Sometimes I feel I just haven't thought about the baby, cared about it enough. I ought to be loving it more.'

COUPLES

Pregnancy is bound to bring about some quite big changes in a couple's relationship, especially if this is your first baby. For some people these changes happen easily, others find it harder to change. Everybody is different.

It's quite common for couples to find themselves having arguments every now and then during pregnancy, however much they are looking forward to the baby. Some of these may be nothing to do with the pregnancy, but others may be caused by one or other partner feeling worried about the future and how they are going to cope. Perhaps the most important thing to realise is that during pregnancy there are

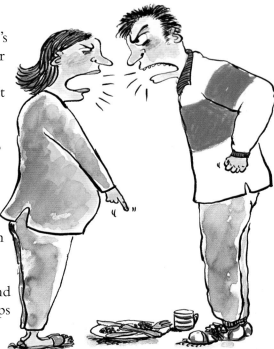

'You hear such a lot and read such a lot in the newspapers about spina bifida and backward children and all that. You can't help but wonder about your own.'

'Now that I've felt it move and I've heard the heartbeat, I feel happier. Early on we worried much more.'

'You've got a bond between you. It's something that belongs to both of you.'

'Sometimes it draws us together and sometimes it sets us apart. When we first found out about the baby, we were on edge. We snapped at each other a lot. Then it got better. We really wanted each other and we were really looking forward to the baby coming. It's up and down.'

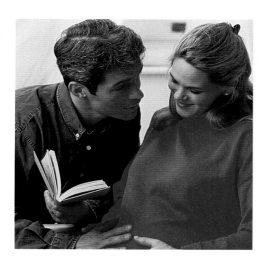

understandable reasons for the odd difficulty between you and also good reasons for feeling closer and more loving.

One practical question you will need to discuss is how you will cope with labour and whether your partner will be there. Many fathers do want to be present at their baby's birth. The chapter on **Labour and birth** (page 89) gives some suggestions on ways in which fathers can help and what it can mean to them to share this experience.

SEX IN PREGNANCY

Many people worry about whether it is safe to have sex during pregnancy. There is no physical reason why you shouldn't continue to have sexual intercourse right through a normal pregnancy, if you wish. It doesn't harm the baby because the penis cannot penetrate beyond the vagina. The muscles of the cervix and a plug of mucus, specially formed in pregnancy, seal off the womb completely.

Later in pregnancy, an orgasm, or even sexual intercourse itself, can set off contractions (known as Braxton Hicks' contractions, see page 90). You will feel the muscles of your womb go hard. There is no need for alarm as this is perfectly normal. If it feels uncomfortable, try your relaxation techniques or just lie quietly till the contractions pass.

If you have had a previous miscarriage, ask your doctor or midwife for advice. Your doctor or midwife will probably advise you to avoid intercourse if you have had heavy bleeding in pregnancy, and you should definitely not have intercourse once the waters have broken (see page 90) since this risks infection in the baby.

While sex is safe for most couples in pregnancy, it may not be all that easy. You will probably need to find different positions. This can be a time to explore and experiment together. The man on top can become very uncomfortable for the woman quite early in pregnancy, not just because of the baby, but because of tender breasts as well. It can also be uncomfortable if the man's penis penetrates too deeply. So it may be better to lie on your sides, either facing or with the man behind. Many couples find that a position in which the woman is on top is most comfortable.

Some couples find making love extra enjoyable during pregnancy while others simply feel that they don't want to have intercourse and prefer to find other ways of being loving or of making love. It's important to talk about your feelings with each other.

FAMILIES AND FRIENDS

In some ways pregnancy is very private, just to do with you and your partner, but there may be a lot of people around you who are also interested and concerned about your baby – parents, sisters, brothers and friends.

People can offer a great deal of help in all sorts of ways and you will probably be very glad of their interest and their support. But sometimes it can feel as if you're being taken over. If so, it can help everyone if you explain gently that

there are some decisions that only you can take and some things that you prefer to do on your own. You may also find that being pregnant puts you on the receiving end of a lot of advice, and perhaps a bit of criticism too. Sometimes the advice is helpful, sometimes not. Sometimes the criticism can really hurt. The important thing is to decide what is right for you. After all, it is your pregnancy and your baby.

'There's the feeling that you're being looked after. Not just by your husband and your parents and the hospital, but by your friends, by everybody. They're there behind you. I suppose they're wrapping me up in cotton wool, but it's still a nice feeling.'

'My mother starts telling me "You must have this for the baby, you must have that", and trying to tell me what I should do. And bringing things like nappy pins and saying "I didn't think you'd remember to get them." It's irritating.'

'We seem to have got a lot closer. We often sit and talk and my mum remembers when I was tiny.'

'It's no good listening to other people. They only tell you about what happened to them. They tell you the bad parts too, not the good.'

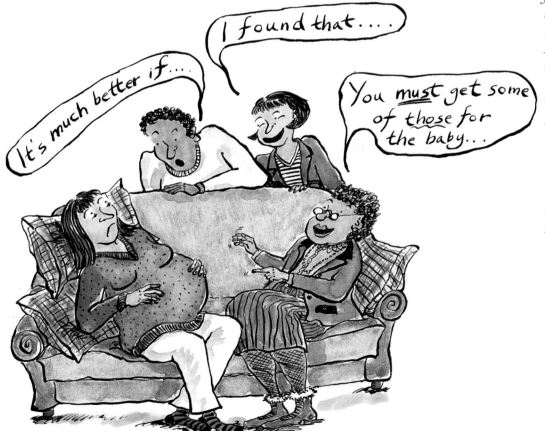

WORK

If you enjoy your work and the company of those you work with, you may have rather mixed feelings when the time comes to stop work before your baby is born. Try to make the most of these few weeks to enjoy doing the things you want to do at your own pace. It is also a good opportunity to make some new friends. You may meet other mothers at your antenatal classes (see pages 64–5) or you may get to know more people living close by, now that you have more time to stop and chat.

You may have decided that you are going to spend some time at home with your baby or you may be planning to return to work, either full or part-time, fairly soon after the birth. If you know that you will be going back to work, or even if you think you might be, you will need to start thinking about who will look after your baby well in advance. It is not always easy to find a satisfactory childcare arrangement and it may take you some time.

Any decision you make about childcare will be determined both by your income and the kind of facilities available locally. You may be lucky enough to have a relative willing to provide care. If not, you should contact your social services department (in Northern Ireland your local Health and Social Services Trust) for a list of registered childminders and nurseries. Few nurseries take babies and prices are usually high. You may also want to consider organising care in your own home, either on your own or sharing with other parents.

Care in your own home does not need to be registered but you should satisfy yourself that your carer is experienced and trained to care for babies. Contact the National Childminding Association or Working for Childcare (see page 143) for more information.

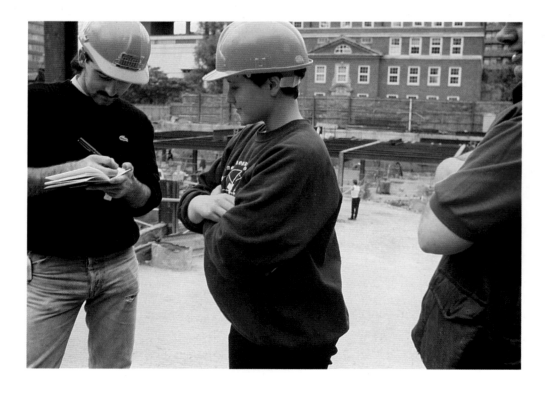

COPING ALONE

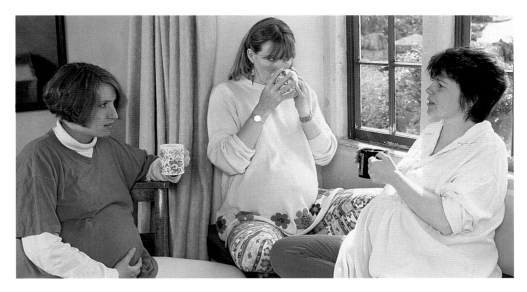

If you're pregnant and on your own it's even more important that there are people with whom you can share your feelings and who can offer you support. Sorting out problems, whether personal or medical, is often difficult when you are by yourself and it's better to find someone to talk to rather than to let things get you down.

You may find it encouraging to meet other mothers who have also gone through pregnancy on their own. Gingerbread (see page 142) is a self-help organisation for one-parent families which has a network of local groups and can offer you information and advice. They will be able to put you in touch with other mothers in a similar situation if you wish.

If money is an immediate concern, read **Rights and benefits** (page 130) for information on what you can claim and your employment rights. Your local social security office, Benefits Agency or local citizens' advice bureau (CAB) will be able to give you more advice. If you have housing problems, contact your local CAB or your local housing advice centre. Ask for the address from your local authority at the town hall (in Northern Ireland contact the

Northern Ireland Housing Executive). The National Council for One Parent Families can also supply information on a range of topics from benefits to maintenance (see page 142). There may be a local support group in your area. Ask your midwife or health visitor.

Don't feel that, just because you don't have a partner, you have to go to antenatal visits and cope with labour on your own. You have as much right as anyone else to be accompanied by the person you choose – a friend, sister, or perhaps your mother. Involve your 'labour partner' in birth classes if you can and let him or her know what you want from them. There may be antenatal classes in your area run especially for single women. Ask your midwife.

Think about how you will manage after the birth. Will there be people around to help and support? If there is no one who can give you support it might help to discuss your situation with a social worker. Your doctor or hospital can refer you or you can contact the social services department of your local council directly.

If you're considering adoption or fostering you should discuss this with a social worker.

'The baby's dad has gone. He wanted the baby at first but when things started to happen he didn't like it, so he's gone. But my mum has been to all my antenatal classes with me and everything, so she knows what's going on.'

'Sometimes I feel really low and think, "Oh God, I'm only 18 and it's for the rest of my life". Every time I go out I've got to get a baby sitter and things.'

'I talked to the hospital social worker about things and she told me all about managing on my own.'

LONE PARENT
HELPLINE
call free on 0800 018 5026

DOMESTIC VIOLENCE

DOMESTIC VIOLENCE

If you need urgent help the following 24-hour helplines are available:

Women's Aid Federation of England
(0345) 023468

In Northern Ireland
(028) 90331818

For Wales see page 143

Rape Crisis
(020) 7837 1600

Refuge
(0990) 995443

One in three women experience domestic violence at some point in their lives. This may take the form of physical, sexual, emotional or psychological abuse. Thirty per cent of this abuse starts in pregnancy and existing abuse may worsen during pregnancy or after birth. Domestic violence should not be tolerated. It risks your health and that of your baby before and after birth.

You can speak in confidence to your GP, midwife, obstetrician, health visitor or social worker. If you wish, they can help you take steps to stop the abuse or to seek refuge. You may prefer to contact one of the organisations listed under domestic violence at the back of this book (page 143), again in confidence.

BENEFITS AVAILABLE IF YOUR PARTNER HAS DIED

- *For advice, you may find the following leaflets produced by the DSS (Social Security Agency in Northern Ireland) helpful:*
  What to Do after Death in England and Wales (D49)
  A Guide to Widow's Benefits (NP45)
  Help from the Social Fund (GL18)
  Which Benefit (FB2)

- *Read Chapter 18 for advice about the following:*
  Income Support   Housing Benefit
  Family Credit   Council Tax
  Child Benefit

- *If you were married and your husband worked, you may be entitled to Widowed Mother's Allowance, based on his National Insurance contributions.*

- *If you weren't married, you will not be classed as a widow and will therefore be dependant on your private arrangements or Income Support or Family Credit, if you work.*

- *If you are very short of money you may be able to get a Funeral Expenses Payment from the Social Fund. It is always worth talking to your undertaker or religious adviser to see if they can help.*

BEREAVEMENT

The death of someone you love can turn your world upside down and is one of the most difficult experiences to endure. This may be harder to cope with if you are pregnant, or just had a baby.

Family and friends can help you by spending time with you if you have been bereaved. A sympathetic arm around the shoulders can express love and support when words are not enough.

Grief is not just one feeling but a whole succession of feelings which take time to get through and which cannot be hurried. If you need help or advice, you can contact your GP or any of the organisations listed on page 142.

IF YOUR PARTNER DIES

If your partner dies during your pregnancy or soon after childbirth you will feel emotionally numb. It is like no other loss. It is not something you get over, more that you learn, eventually, to live with.

Don't be afraid to lean on family and friends. If your partner was going to be with you at the birth you will need to think about who will be with you instead. Try to choose someone who knows you very well.

Financially, you may need urgent advice and support. You can get the leaflets suggested (see box) from your local social security office/Benefits Agency.

As well as speaking to friends, family and social services, you may like to contact WIDWODS, a small support group set up by young widows (see page 142).

6 Mainly for men

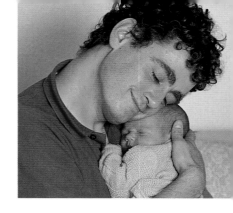

Some pregnancies have been planned for months or years, but many are unexpected. Either way, you'll probably feel pretty mixed up. A baby means new responsibilities which, whatever your age, you may feel unready for.

YOUR FEELINGS ABOUT PREGNANCY

Your partner may have similar feelings. It's normal for both of you to feel like this. Your first pregnancy is a very important event. It will change your life and change can be frightening even if it's something you've been looking forward to. Money problems may be nagging at you – the loss of an income for a while, extra expenses for the baby and, if your partner returns to work, the cost of childcare. You may be worrying that your home isn't right or that you'll feel obliged to stay in a job you don't like. (It might help to look at the **Rights and benefits** section on page 130 and start planning ahead.)

Some men feel left out. Your partner's attention will be on what's happening inside her and she may want you to pay a lot more attention to her needs than usual. You may not have realised how much you relied on her to make you feel cared for and now that her attention is elsewhere you may feel quite lonely. Your loneliness may be increased if your partner doesn't want to make love, although some women find sex more enjoyable than ever. It varies from person to person. There's

usually no medical reason to avoid sex, but keep in mind:

- her breasts in the early weeks may be extremely painful;

- if there's any bleeding or pain avoid intercourse (and consult your doctor);

- make sure your partner is comfortable – you may need to try different positions as the pregnancy progresses.

If she's not interested in sex, try to find other ways of being close, but do talk about it. If she feels that you're trying to persuade her to do something she doesn't want, she may withdraw completely leaving both of you lonely.

Some men find it hard to make love during pregnancy. They feel strange doing it with 'someone else there' or may find their partner's changing shape disturbing. This is one situation when it helps to be careful what you say. Your partner may well feel uneasy about her changing body and may be very hurt if she thinks that you don't like it either.

'When the test was positive, I felt really excited, on a real high. We couldn't wait to tell everyone.'

(A FATHER)

'It was a shock at first, but now I'm getting used to the idea. We didn't plan it, but there's no problem with that. If it had been three years ago, when we first started living together, obviously it would have been a lot worse financially. That's the main factor.'

(A FATHER)

47

TALK ABOUT IT

'She became very absorbed in her own body, separate. I felt lonely and frightened of not doing the right thing.'

(A FATHER)

'My worries are to do with making sure that she's happy and comfortable and that.'

(A FATHER)

Confide in friends who are already fathers and will know what you're going through. You may want to protect your partner from your worries but she will almost certainly sense your concern. The more you keep it to yourself, the more she'll feel that you're moving away from her – just when she badly needs you to be there. If you're giving her the support she needs, then there's no need to leave your feelings out of the picture.

PHYSICAL FEELINGS

Believe it or not, men can get symptoms of pregnancy too! The most commonly reported ones are sleeplessness, indigestion and nausea. They are probably caused by stress, but are no less uncomfortable for that.

SUPPORTING YOUR PARTNER

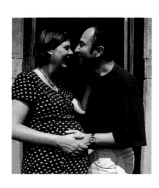

'My wife one day couldn't stand the smell of me. I tried every different kind of soap, but it made no difference. In the end I asked the doctor about it.'

(A FATHER)

'I am happy to be involved. I want to know what she has to do. I like to feel involved, contributing to this, not just starting it.'

(A FATHER)

Something amazing is happening inside your partner's body. The closer you can get to her, the more you'll be able to share this experience. But at times closeness will seem impossible.

In the early weeks she may be prickly and irritable about the slightest things. Certain smells and tastes may make her nauseous. She may want only to sleep.

In the middle months you'll probably find that much of her energy returns and she may resent being treated 'like china'.

Towards the end the weight of the baby may drag her down. The tiredness and irritability of the early weeks often returns and she may start feeling quite frightened of the birth and be lonely without the company of friends at work.

If your partner is anxious, encourage her to talk about it. Many women are more used to listening than being listened to, so it may take a while before she feels able to open up. Be patient – the better you can learn to support each other now, the stronger your relationship will be when the baby arrives.

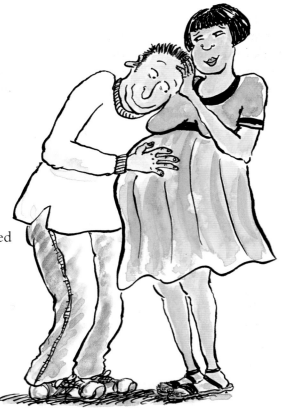

PRACTICAL SUPPORT

Your partner may be used to doing most of the housework as well as going out to work. If she continues to do all this work she'll tire herself out. Now is the time to start sharing the housework if you don't already do so. There are two areas where you can really help:

- cooking – in the early months the smell may put her off and if you cook she's more likely to eat what she needs;

- carrying heavy shopping can put a lot of strain on her back, so try to do the shopping yourself or together.

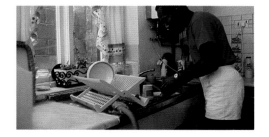

A FRIEND IN NEED

Pregnancy can be frightening so it will help if she knows that she's not alone. Start by reading the rest of this book with her so that you're both well informed. Some of the basic health advice is just as important for you as it is for her.

- Good eating is much easier if you're doing it together, so read pages 8-12 and start picking up the food habits you'll want to pass on to your child.

- Cigarette smoke is dangerous for babies. If you are a smoker read page 13 on how to stop.

- If you continue to smoke, don't smoke near your partner, don't offer her cigarettes and don't leave your cigarettes lying around.

- Go with her to the doctor if she's worried, or be sure to talk it through when she gets home.

- Be there if she has a scan (see page 56) and see your baby on the screen.

- If she needs to have extra tests (see pages 53-9) your support is especially important.

- Find out about antenatal classes for couples, or fathers' evenings at the hospital (see pages 64-5). The more you know about labour, the more you'll be able to help.

- Most men stay with their partners during labour but it's important that you're both happy about it. If you prefer not to be present, talk to your partner. You may be able to think of a friend or relative who could accompany her instead.

- Talk about what you both expect in labour (see page 34).

- Talk about the birth plan (see page 38). Fill it in together so you know what she wants and how you can help her achieve it. Support her if she changes her mind during labour. Be flexible.

- During labour she'll be far too involved with what's happening inside to pay much attention to the people around her. You can be her guide and interpreter.

PATERNITY LEAVE

Speak to your Human Resources department or your boss about the paternity leave entitlement in your company. More employers are now realising that partners need time off work when they have a new baby.

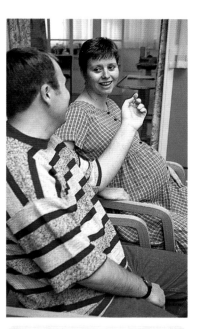

THE BIRTH — BEING PREPARED

A checklist for the final weeks

- *Make sure your partner can contact you at all times.*

- *Decide how you'll get to the hospital (if you're having a hospital birth).*

- *If you're using your own car, make sure it works, has petrol and do a trial run to see how long it takes.*

- *Remember to pack a bag for yourself including snacks, a camera and film, and change for the telephone.*

'From time to time I became angry. She was complaining too much, but millions of women become pregnant don't they?'

(A FATHER)

BECOMING A FATHER

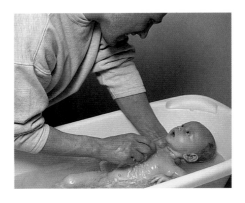

Watching your baby coming into the world is the most incredible experience. The midwives will give you the baby to hold. Some men feel afraid of hurting such a tiny creature. Don't be. Hold the baby close to your body. Feel the softness of the head against your cheek.

Many fathers experience very strong emotions; some cry. It can be very difficult to go home and rest after such an intense experience, so think through what your needs might be at this time. You may need to tell someone all about the birth before you can rest, but then sleep if you can. You need to recover from the birth too and, when the baby comes home (if the birth took place in hospital), you can expect broken nights for some time to come.

BRINGING THEM HOME

You may find that relatives and friends are able to help in the early days so that your partner can rest and feed your baby. This is especially necessary after a difficult birth. However, you may live far from relatives and she may only have you. It's a good idea to have a week or so off work if you can. Think about the following:

- too many visitors may exhaust her and interfere with this special time when you are learning about being parents and a family;

- you could look after the baby so she can get a good rest each day;

- take over the basic housework, but don't feel you must keep the place spotless – no one should expect it;

- try to use this time to get to know your baby – you could learn to change nappies and bath your baby as well as cuddling and playing with him or her; if your partner is breastfeeding you could bring her a snack and a drink while she feeds the baby; if bottle feeding, you could sterilise and make up the bottles (see page 73) and share the feeding;

- when you go back to work you may have to make up for her lost earnings, but keep overtime to a minimum – you will want to continue learning about your baby and being there so you can watch your child grow and develop;

- be considerate about sex – it may take many weeks or months before she stops feeling sore; you could discuss other ways of showing your love for each other until intercourse is comfortable.

FEELING LOW

Some mothers become depressed and need a lot of extra support, both practical and emotional (see **The baby blues and postnatal depression,** page 117). You may also get depressed. Your partner is facing the biggest changes but that doesn't mean that you should ignore your own feelings. You need support too. Keep talking and listening to each other, talk to friends too, and be patient – life will get easier in time.

7 Antenatal care and antenatal classes

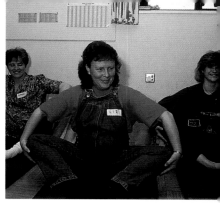

Throughout your pregnancy you will have regular care, either at a hospital antenatal clinic or with your own GP or community midwife. This is to check that you and the baby are well and so that any problems can be picked up as early as possible. This is the time to get answers to any questions or worries and to discuss plans for your baby's birth.

THE FIRST VISIT

Most women have their first, and longest, antenatal check-up around the 8th to 12th week of pregnancy. The earlier you go the better. You should allow plenty of time as you will probably see a midwife and a doctor, and may be offered an ultrasound scan.

QUESTIONS

You can expect a lot of questions on your health, on any illnesses and operations you have had, and on any previous pregnancies or miscarriages. You will be asked for any information you have on your own family and your partner's family (whether there are twins on your side or any inherited illness, for example). You will also be asked about your ethnic origin. This is because certain inherited conditions that need attention in early pregnancy are more common in some ethnic groups.

There may also be questions about your work or your partner's work and what kind of accommodation you live in, to see if there is anything about your circumstances that might affect your pregnancy.

All this information will help to build up a picture of you and your pregnancy so that any special risks can be spotted and support provided.

The midwife or doctor will want to know the date of the first day of your last period, to work out when the baby is due. You will probably want to ask a lot of questions yourself. This is a good opportunity and it often helps if you can write down what you want to say in advance, as it's easy to forget once you are there. It's important to find out what you want to know and to express your own feelings and preferences.

Remember that, if you're working, you have the right to paid time off for your antenatal care (see page 139).

If you don't speak English, ask a friend who does to come with you and interpret, or telephone your clinic so that an interpreter can be arranged for when you have an appointment.

LET YOUR MIDWIFE OR DOCTOR KNOW IF:

- *there were any complications in a previous pregnancy or delivery, such as pre-eclampsia or premature delivery;*

- *you are being treated for a chronic disease such as diabetes or high blood pressure;*

- *you, or anyone in your family, have previously had a baby with an abnormality, for example spina bifida, or there is a family history of an inherited disease such as thalassaemia or cystic fibrosis.*

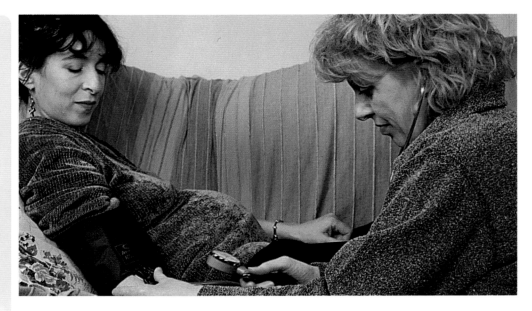

WEIGHT

You'll be weighed. From now on, your weight gain will probably be checked regularly, although this is not done everywhere. Most women put on between 10–12.5 kg (22–28 lbs) in pregnancy, most of it after the 20th week. Read pages 8-12 on what to eat in pregnancy, and take regular exercise. Much of the extra weight is due to the baby growing, but your body will also be storing fat ready to make breast milk after the birth.

HEIGHT

Your height will be recorded on the first visit because it is a rough guide to the size of your pelvis. Some small women have small pelvises and although they often have small babies they may need to discuss their baby's delivery with their doctor or midwife.

GENERAL PHYSICAL EXAMINATION

The doctor will check your heart and lungs and make sure your general health is good.

URINE

You will be asked to give a sample of urine each time you visit. This will be checked for a number of things including:

- **sugar** – pregnant women may have sugar in their urine from time to time but, if it is found repeatedly, you will be checked for diabetes (some women develop a type of diabetes in pregnancy known as 'gestational diabetes' which can be controlled during pregnancy usually by a change of diet and, possibly, insulin; the condition usually disappears once the baby is born);

- **protein**, or 'albumin', in your urine may show that there is an infection that needs to be treated; it may also be a sign of pregnancy-induced hypertension (see **High blood pressure and pre-eclampsia** on page 84).

BLOOD PRESSURE

Your blood pressure will be taken at every antenatal visit. A rise in blood pressure later in pregnancy could be a sign of pre-eclampsia (see page 84).

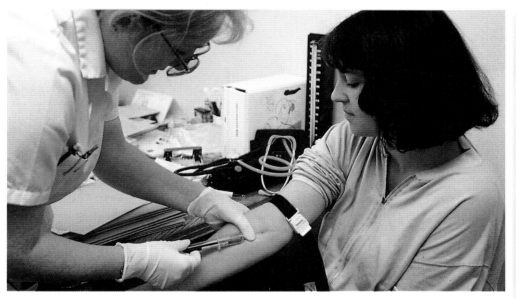

TESTS

A number of tests will be offered at your first visit, and some of these will be repeated at later visits. You are under no obligation to have any test, although they are all done to help make your pregnancy safer or to help assess the well-being of your baby. Discuss the reasons for tests with your midwife or doctor so that you can make an informed choice about whether or not to have them. Ask to have the results explained to you if you do decide to go ahead.

BLOOD TESTS

You will be offered a blood test which will check:

- **your blood group**;

- **whether your blood is rhesus negative or positive** – a few mothers are rhesus negative (usually this is not a worry for the first pregnancy. Some rhesus negative mothers will need an injection after the birth of their first baby to protect their next baby from anaemia.; in some units, rhesus negative mothers are given injections called 'anti-D' at 28 and 34 weeks as well as after the birth of their baby – this is quite safe and is done to make sure that the blood of future babies is not affected by rhesus disease – see page 110);

- **whether you are anaemic** – if you are, you will probably be given iron and folic acid tablets to take (anaemia makes you tired and less able to cope with losing blood at delivery);

- **your immunity to rubella** (German measles) – if you get rubella in early pregnancy, it can seriously damage your unborn baby and if you are not immune to rubella and come into contact with it, blood tests will show whether you have been infected; if so, you'll be offered the option of ending your pregnancy after discussing the possible problems your baby might have;

- **for syphilis** – it is vital to detect and treat any woman who has this sexually transmitted infection as early as possible;

- **for hepatitis B** – this is a virus which causes liver disease and may infect the baby if you are a carrier of the virus or are infected during pregnancy (the baby can be immunised at birth to prevent infection (see page 101), so most units will routinely offer a test to check if you are carrying the virus).

IF YOU ARE FOUND TO BE HIV POSITIVE,

or already know that you are, your doctor will need to discuss the management of your pregnancy and delivery with you.

- *There is a 15% chance of your baby being infected.*

- *Treatment may reduce the risk of transmitting HIV from you to the baby.*

- *Your baby will be tested for HIV at birth and at intervals for up to two years. If the baby is found to be HIV infected, paediatricians will be able to anticipate certain illnesses which occur in infected babies, and so treat them early. All babies born to HIV positive mothers will appear to be HIV positive at birth but many later test negative because antibodies passed to them by their mothers disappear.*

- *You will be advised not to breastfeed because HIV can be transmitted to your baby in this way.*

- *Your labour will be managed to reduce the risk of infection to your baby.*

HIV BLOOD TEST

HIV is the virus that causes AIDS. You won't be tested routinely for HIV infection, but some hospitals are carrying out unlinked anonymous surveys to try to find out just how widespread HIV is in the population. If your hospital is one of these, then leaflets and posters explaining the survey should be on display.

Anonymous testing involves testing some of the blood from the routine checks described above, for HIV antibodies. All specimens have any details which could identify the woman permanently removed before testing so that there is no possibility that your result can be traced back to you. You can ask for your specimen to be excluded from the survey if you wish. You can be sure that the survey will not affect your antenatal care in any way.

In some hospitals (usually those in inner city areas) the prevalence of HIV has been found to be higher than that of the general population through this anonymous testing. A named confidential HIV test is being offered to all women in some of these units, so that interventions known to decrease the risk of the baby being infected can be offered to infected women (see box).

If you think that you may have been at risk of getting HIV, ask your doctor or midwife for the opportunity to discuss HIV testing and counselling. If you're HIV positive, you can talk to someone at Positively Women, an organisation concerned with women and HIV and AIDS (see page 143).

SICKLE CELL DISEASE AND THALASSAEMIA

Sickle cell disease is a blood condition that mainly affects people of African and West Indian origin and, less often, people from India, the Middle East and Mediterranean. Thalassaemia, another blood condition, mainly affects people of Mediterranean and Asian origin. If you, your partner, or your parents originally come from these parts of the world, you'll probably be offered a blood test to find out whether you are a carrier. It is possible for either you or your partner to be a carrier

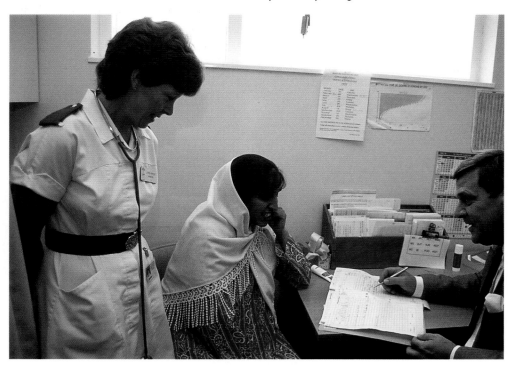

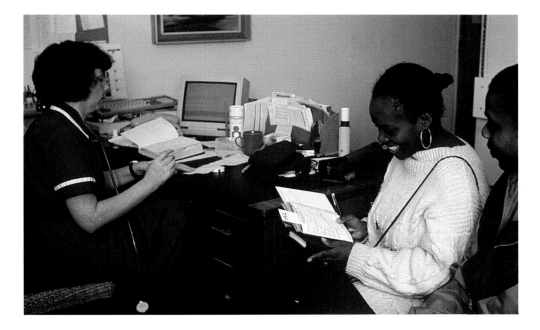

without it affecting your baby at all. But if both of you are carriers, or if either of you suffer from the disease yourself, you should discuss the implications for the baby with your doctor or midwife. Or contact the Sickle Cell Society or the UK Thalassaemia Society (see page 143).

INTERNAL EXAMINATION

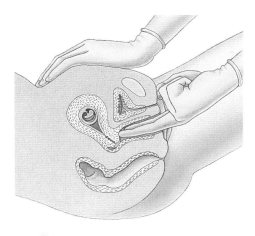

Occasionally, the doctor might consider it necessary to do an internal examination. Discuss the reasons for this with the doctor. By putting one or two fingers inside your vagina and pressing the other hand on your abdomen, your doctor can judge the age of your baby. Most doctors prefer to use an ultrasound scan for this purpose (see page 56) either at the first or a later visit.

CERVICAL SMEAR

You will be offered a cervical smear test now if you haven't had one in the last three years. The test detects early changes in the cervix (the neck of the womb) which could later lead to cancer if left untreated. By sliding an instrument called a speculum into your vagina, the doctor can look at your cervix. A smear is then taken from the surface of the cervix and will be examined under a microscope. The test may feel a bit uncomfortable but it is not painful and won't harm the growing baby.

HERPES

If you, or your partner, have ever had genital herpes, or you get your first attack of genital blisters or ulcers during your pregnancy, let your doctor or midwife know. This is important because herpes can be dangerous for your newborn baby and he or she may need treatment (see page 18).

LATER VISITS

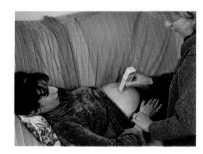

Later visits are usually shorter. Your urine and blood pressure, and often your weight, will be checked. Your abdomen will be felt to check the baby's position and growth. And the doctor or midwife will listen to your baby's heartbeat. You can also ask questions or talk about anything that is worrying you. Talking is as much a part of antenatal care as all the tests and examinations.

From now on, antenatal checks will usually be every four weeks until 28 weeks, every two weeks until 36 weeks, and then every week until the baby is born. If your pregnancy is uncomplicated, you may be offered the option of less frequent antenatal appointments. If you can't keep an antenatal appointment, let the clinic, GP or midwife know, and make another appointment.

ULTRASOUND SCAN

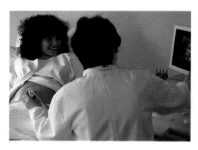

This test uses sound waves to build up a picture of the baby in the womb. Most hospitals will offer women at least one ultrasound scan during their pregnancy. An ultrasound scan can be used to:

- check the baby's measurements – this gives a better idea of the baby's age and can help decide when your baby is likely to be born – this can be useful if you are unsure about the date of your last period or if your menstrual cycle is long, short or irregular; your due date may be adjusted according to ultrasound measurements;

- check whether you are carrying more than one baby;

- detect some abnormalities, particularly in the baby's head or spine;

- show the position of the baby and the placenta – in some cases, for example where the placenta is low in late pregnancy, special care may be needed at delivery or a Caesarean section may be advised;

- check that the baby is growing and developing normally (this is particularly important if you are carrying twins or more).

The scan is completely painless, has no known serious side-effects on mothers or their babies (although research is continuing), and can be carried out at any stage of pregnancy. Most hospitals scan all women at 18 to 20 weeks to check for certain abnormalities.

You will probably be asked to drink a lot of fluid before you have the scan. A full bladder pushes your womb up and this gives a better picture. You then lie on your back and some jelly is put on your abdomen. An instrument is passed backwards and forwards over your skin and high-frequency sound is beamed through your abdomen into the womb. The sound is reflected back and creates a picture which is shown on a TV screen. It can be very exciting to see a picture of your own baby before birth, often moving about inside.

Ask for the picture to be explained to you if you can't make it out. It may be possible for your partner to come with you and see the scan. Many couples feel that this helps to make the baby real for them both. Ask if it's possible to have a copy of the picture. (There may be a small charge for this.)

If you feel doubtful about having a scan, talk it over with your GP, midwife or obstetrician.

TESTS TO DETECT ABNORMALITIES IN THE BABY

It is important to realise that no test can guarantee that your baby will be born without abnormality. No test is 100% accurate and some abnormalities may remain undetected.

The tests below are designed to detect **structural abnormalities** like spina bifida or **genetic disorders** like Down's syndrome. Down's syndrome is caused by an abnormal number of chromosomes. Chromosomes are the structures within every cell of a person's body which carry the individual genetic code or recipe to make that person. Conditions like cystic fibrosis and achondroplasia (dwarfism) are caused by abnormalities within the chromosomes (so causing a 'mistake' in the recipe). Talk to your midwife, GP or obstetrician about the tests mentioned below as they are not available in all hospitals.

When you are deciding whether or not to have a test, think what you might do if the test suggests that your baby has an abnormality. If a screening test (**serum screen** or **nuchal translucency**) suggests a 'high' risk of genetic abnormality, you will be offered **amniocentesis** or **chorionic villus sampling** (**CVS**). Since these carry a risk of miscarriage, you may decide not to have these tests or even a screening test if you would choose to continue with the pregnancy. Having a test, however, may reassure you that your baby is likely to be born healthy, allow you to consider the termination of an affected baby or give you time to prepare for the arrival of a baby with special needs. Discuss the issues with your partner, midwife, doctor and friends.

ULTRASOUND (see also page 56)

Since ultrasound provides an image of the baby in the womb, it detects structural abnormalities, particularly of the spine and head. Recently, however, it has been found to be useful in screening for Down's syndrome and some other abnormalities of chromosome number. Several research studies have shown that the thickness of the 'nuchal fold' at the back of the baby's neck is related to the risk of Down's syndrome. An ultrasound scan at 10 to 13 weeks enables a measurement to be taken. This measurement then allows a risk factor to be calculated. The nuchal translucency scan is not widely available at present but it is becoming more so. It cannot be used to assess the risk of Down's syndrome in twin pregnancies.

ALPHA-FETOPROTEIN (AFP) TEST

This test is performed at about 15 to 20 weeks to find out the level of alpha-fetoprotein (AFP) in your blood. This protein is made by your baby and passes into your blood during pregnancy. High levels are associated with spina bifida and so an ultrasound scan will then be offered to check for this. High levels may be seen in normal pregnancy and also in twin pregnancy. Low levels of AFP are associated with Down's syndrome pregnancies. Ultrasound and amniocentesis will then be suggested to achieve a diagnosis.

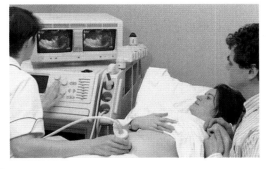

Some hospitals routinely offer the AFP test to all women; others don't, or restrict the test to older women since the risk of Down's syndrome, and some other abnormalities of chromosome number, increases with age.

IF A TEST DETECTS AN ABNORMALITY,

*you may like to contact the appropriate organisation (see page 141–3) for further information. They may be able to put you in touch with parents who have decided to continue with a pregnancy in which an abnormality has been detected. **ARC** (Antenatal Results and Choices; see page 142) will offer support and information if you are considering termination for abnormality.*

SERUM SCREENING

This is the term used for a test of the mother's blood which screens for Down's syndrome. It combines the AFP result (and so gives information about the risk of spina bifida) with the measurement of other blood chemicals to give the relative risk of having a baby with Down's syndrome. There are various tests available ('double test', 'triple plus test', etc.) which differ slightly from each other, but they are all types of serum screening. They are not helpful in twin or other multiple pregnancies.

Some units give the result as 'screen negative' or 'screen positive'. A negative result means that Down's syndrome is unlikely. A positive result means that Down's syndrome is more likely. An amniocentesis will be suggested to give more information. Other units give a numerical result, for example 1:250 risk of Down's syndrome. You may like to compare this risk to that for your age (about 1:900 at 30) or to the risk of miscarriage with amniocentesis (about 1:100). Your doctor or midwife will explain the significance of the result to you. If the test is not available locally on the NHS, you may be able to obtain a test privately.

AMNIOCENTESIS

This test may be offered from 14 weeks of pregnancy:

- to women who have an AFP, serum screening or nuchal translucency scan result which indicates an increased risk of Down's syndrome;

- when an ultrasound scan detects an abnormality which is associated with a genetic disorder;

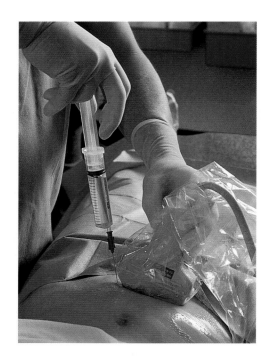

- when a woman's past or family history suggests that there may be a risk of her baby having a genetic disorder such as Down's syndrome.

An ultrasound scan is performed to check the position of the baby and placenta. Whilst continuing to scan with the ultrasound probe, a fine needle is passed through the wall of the abdomen into the amniotic fluid which surrounds the baby. A small sample of this fluid is drawn off and sent to the laboratory for testing. Most women feel only mild discomfort.

Within the fluid are cells which contain the same chromosomes as the baby. Looking at these chromosomes is a complex process which is why the results take up to three weeks. This test will reveal your baby's sex. Tell your doctor whether or not you want to know what it is. Some disorders such as haemophilia and muscular dystrophy are only found in boys (although girls may carry the disorder in their chromosomes and pass it on to their sons). Tell your doctor if these or other genetic disorders run in your family as it may then be important to know your baby's sex.

Amniocentesis is associated with a 0.5–1% risk of miscarriage. At most, one test in a hundred will result in pregnancy loss. When deciding whether or not to go ahead with this test try to balance the risk of miscarriage against the value of the result to you. Remember that a normal result only reassures you about the number of chromosomes unless specific tests for disorders such as cystic fibrosis have been done.

CHORIONIC VILLUS SAMPLING (CVS)

This test is usually only available in large hospitals but smaller units are able to refer to these units if necessary. It tests for genetic disorders. It does not give information about spina bifida.

CVS can be carried out earlier than amniocentesis at around ten weeks but may carry a slightly higher risk of miscarriage, at about 1%. CVS before ten weeks has been associated with a slightly increased risk of limb deformities. Women at risk of having a child with an inherited disorder such as cystic fibrosis or muscular dystrophy may accept the increased risk of miscarriage in order to obtain an earlier diagnosis.

The test takes 10 to 20 minutes and may be a little uncomfortable. Using ultrasound as a guide, a fine needle is passed through the woman's abdomen, or sometimes a fine tube through the vagina and cervix, into the womb. A tiny piece of the developing placenta, known as chorionic tissue, is withdrawn. Again, the chromosomes in the cells of this tissue are looked at. The results take up to two weeks.

If you feel the test would be helpful, talk over the matter carefully with your GP or midwife early in your pregnancy or before conception, as well as with your partner or a close friend. You can also contact your regional genetic centre direct (telephone the Genetic Interest Group for details of your nearest centre, see page 142).

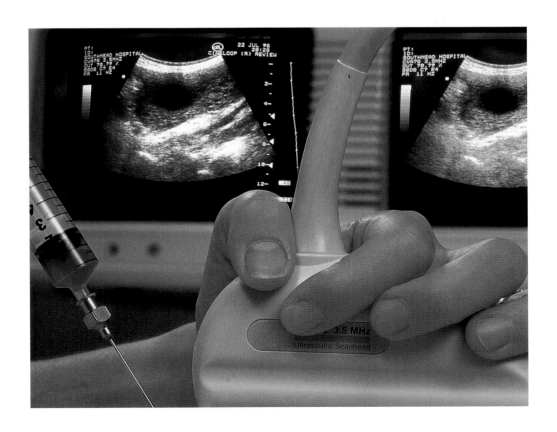

MAKING THE MOST OF ANTENATAL CARE

'There were some things that really annoyed me – the gowns, and the lavatories, and one midwife who called everyone "sweetie". But there were other things I wouldn't have missed – like hearing my baby's heart beating, and well, just knowing she was all right. Knowing I was all right too, come to that.'

'I think it's up to you to make the most of it. You can find out a lot, but you have to ask. When your blood pressure's taken, you have to say, "Is that all right?". Then they'll tell you. And if it's not all right, you have to ask why not, and talk about it. It's the same for everything. It's not being a nuisance, it's being interested. I think the staff like it if you're interested.'

If you have a disability which means that you have special requirements for your antenatal appointments or for labour, let your midwife know so that arrangements can be made in advance.

Having regular antenatal care is important for your health and the health of your baby. However, sometimes antenatal visits can seem quite an effort. If the clinic is busy or short-staffed you may have to wait a long time and, if you have small children with you, this can be very exhausting. By increasing the number of women that are cared for by their GP and community midwife, antenatal care should become more convenient. Try to plan ahead to make your visits easier and come prepared to wait. Here are some suggestions.

- In some clinics you can buy refreshments. If not, take a snack with you if you are likely to get hungry.

- Write a list of any questions you want to ask and take it with you to remind you. Make sure you get answers to your questions or the opportunity to discuss any worries. Sometimes this can take quite a lot of determination.

- If your partner is free he may be able to go with you. He'll be able to support you in discussing any worries or in finding out what you want to know. It will also help him to feel more involved in your pregnancy.

- If you regularly wait for long periods at your clinic, bring this to the attention of the hospital management. They have a responsibility to ensure that Patient's Charter standards are met.

YOUR ANTENATAL NOTES

At your first antenatal visit, your doctor or midwife will enter your details in a record book and add to them at each visit. Many hospitals ask women to look after these notes themselves. Other hospitals keep the notes and give you a card which records your details. Take your notes or card with you wherever you go. Then, if you need medical attention while you are away from home, you will have the information that's needed with you.

The page opposite gives a sample of the information your card or notes may contain, as each clinic has its own system. Always ask your doctor or midwife about anything on your card which you would like to have explained.

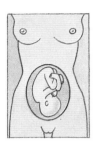

R.O.L. or R.O.T.   L.O.P

L.O.A.

L.O.L.
or
L.O.T   R.O.A.   R.O.P.

POSITION

The above abbreviations are used to describe the way the baby is lying – facing sideways, for example, or frontwards or backwards. Ask your midwife to explain the way your baby is lying.

RELATION TO BRIM

At the end of pregnancy your baby's head (or bottom, or feet if it is in the breech position) will start to move into your pelvis. Doctors and midwives 'divide' the baby's head into 'fifths' and describe how far it has moved down into the pelvis by judging how many 'fifths' of the head they can feel above the brim (the bone at the front).

They may say that the head is 'engaged' – this is when $2/5$ or less of the baby's head can be 'felt' (palpated) above the brim. This may not happen until you are in labour. If all of the baby's head can be felt above the brim, this is described as 'free' or $5/5$.

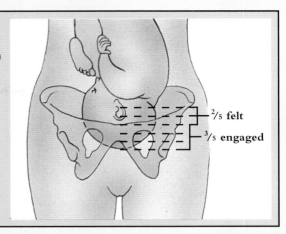

$2/5$ felt

$3/5$ engaged

BLOOD PRESSURE (BP)
This usually stays at about the same level throughout pregnancy. If it goes up a lot in the last half of pregnancy, it may be a sign of pre-eclampsia which can be dangerous for you and your baby (see page 84).

FETAL HEART
'FHH' or just 'H' means 'foetal heart heard'. 'FMF' means 'foetal movement felt'.

OEDEMA
This is another word for swelling, most often of the feet and hands. Usually it is nothing to worry about, but tell your doctor or midwife if it suddenly gets worse as this may be a sign of pre-eclampsia (see page 84).

Hb
This stands for 'haemoglobin'. It is tested in your blood sample to check you are not anaemic.

DATE	WEEKS	WEIGHT	URINE ALB SUGAR	BP	HEIGHT FUNDUS	PRESENTATION AND POSITION	RELATION OF PP TO BRIM	FH	OEDEMA	Hb	NEXT	SIGN.	NOTES
15/6/99	13	58 kg	Nil	110/60	15	-	-	-	-	12.0	20/7	CS	u/s arranged for 17/7 to check maturity
20/7/99	18	59.2 kg	Nil	125/60	18-20	-	-	FMF	-	-	21/8	CS	
21/8/99	22	61 kg	Nil	135/65	20	-	-	-	-	-	18/9	CS	taking iron
18/9/99	26+	64 kg	Nil	125/75	24-26	-	-	H	-	11.2	28/10	CS	
28/10/99	30	66 kg	Nil	125/70	30	ceph	5/5	FHH	-	-	27/11	CS	Mat B1 given, Hb taken
27/11/99	34	-	Nil	115/75	34	ceph	4/5	FHH	-	11.0	15/12	CS	

DATE
This is the date of your antenatal visit.

WEEKS
This refers to the length of your pregnancy in weeks from the date of your last menstrual period.

PRESENTATION
This refers to which way up the baby is. Up to about 30 weeks, the baby moves about a lot. Then it usually settles into its head downward position, ready to be born head first. This is recorded as 'Vx' (vertex) or 'C' or 'ceph' (cephalic). Both words mean the top of the head. If your baby stays with its bottom downwards, this is a breech ('Br') presentation. 'PP' means presenting part, that is the bit of the baby that is coming first. 'Tr' (transverse) means your baby is lying across your tummy.

URINE
These are the results of your urine tests for protein and sugar. '+' or 'Tr' means a quantity (or trace) has been found. 'Alb' stands for 'albumin', a name for one of the proteins detected in urine. 'Nil' or a tick or 'NAD' all mean the same: nothing abnormal discovered. 'Ketones' may be found if you have not eaten recently or have been vomiting.

HEIGHT OF FUNDUS
By gently pressing on your abdomen, the doctor or midwife can feel your womb. Early in pregnancy the top of the womb, or 'fundus', can be felt low down, below your navel. Towards the end it is well up above your navel, just under your breasts. So the height of the fundus is a guide to how many weeks pregnant you are. This column gives the length of your pregnancy, in weeks, estimated according to the position of the fundus. The figure should be roughly the same as the figure in the 'weeks' column. If there's a big difference (say, more than two weeks), ask your doctor about it. Sometimes the height of the fundus may be measured with a tape measure and the result entered on your card in centimetres.

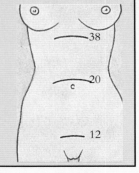

38

20

12

WHO'S WHO

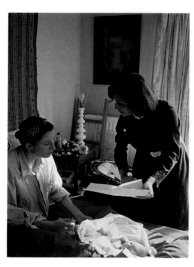

Many mothers would like to be able to get to know the people who care for them during pregnancy and the birth of their baby. The NHS is now working to achieve this. However, you may still find that you see a number of different carers. Professionals should, of course, introduce themselves and explain what they do but, if they forget, don't hesitate to ask. It may help to make a note of who you have seen and what they have said in case you need to discuss any point later on. Below are the people you're most likely to meet. Some may have students with them who are being trained and you will be asked if you mind them being present.

- **A midwife** is specially trained to care for mothers and babies throughout normal pregnancy, labour and after the birth, and therefore provides all care for the majority of women at home or in hospital. Increasingly, midwives will be working both in hospital and in the community so that they can provide better continuity of care. You should know the name of the midwife who is responsible for your midwifery care.

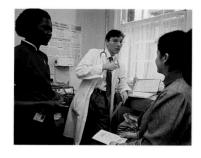

- **A hospital midwife** will probably see you each time you go to a hospital antenatal clinic. A midwife will look after you during labour and will probably deliver your baby, if your delivery is normal. If any complications develop during your pregnancy or delivery, a doctor will become more closely involved with your care. You and your baby will be cared for by midwives on the postnatal ward until you go home. You will probably also meet student midwives and student doctors.

- **A community midwife** will probably get to know you before your baby is born and will visit you at home, after you leave hospital during the early weeks. Community midwives are sometimes attached to GPs' practices and may be involved in giving antenatal care. They are also involved in delivering babies in community and GP or midwife units and are responsible for home deliveries. Some community midwives also accompany women into the hospital maternity unit to be with them for the birth.

- **Your general practitioner (GP)** can help you to plan your antenatal care. This may be given at the hospital, but it is quite often shared with the GP. Sometimes the GP may be responsible for all your antenatal care and in some areas may be responsible for your care in hospital. If you have your baby in a GP or midwife unit or at home, your GP may be involved in your baby's birth. If your baby is born in hospital, your GP will be notified of your baby's birth and will arrange to see you soon after you return home. Don't forget to register your baby with your GP.

- **An obstetrician** is a doctor specialising in the care of women during pregnancy, labour and soon after the birth. If you are having a hospital birth you will usually be under the care of a consultant and the doctors on his or her own team, together with other professionals such as midwives. In some hospitals you will routinely see an obstetrician; in others, your midwife or GP will refer you for an appointment if they have a particular concern such as previous complications of pregnancy or labour or chronic illness. If everything is straightforward, a midwife will usually deliver your baby. You should ask to see your consultant if you wish to discuss any matter you think is important.

- **A paediatrician** is a doctor specialising in the care of babies and children. The paediatrician may check your baby after the birth to make sure all is well and will be present when your baby is born if you have had a difficult labour. If your baby should have any problems, you will be able to talk this over with the paediatrician. If your baby is born at home or your stay in hospital is short, you may not see a paediatrician at all. Your GP can check that all is well with you and your baby.

- **An obstetric physiotherapist** is specially trained to help you cope with the physical changes of pregnancy, childbirth and afterwards. Some attend antenatal classes and teach antenatal exercises, relaxation and breathing, active positions and other ways you can help yourself during pregnancy and labour. Afterwards, they advise on postnatal exercises to tone up your muscles again. When no obstetric physiotherapist is available your midwife can help you with these exercises.

- **Health visitors** are specially trained nurses concerned with the health of the whole family. You may meet yours before the birth of your baby. The health visitor will contact you to arrange a home visit when your baby is ten days old to offer help and support. You may continue to see your health visitor either at home, or at your Child Health Clinic, health centre or GP's surgery, depending on where they are based.

- **Dietitians** are available to advise you on healthy eating or if you need to follow a special diet such as that recommended for women with gestational diabetes.

RESEARCH

You may be asked to participate in a research project during your antenatal care, labour or postnatally. This may involve a new treatment or be to find out your opinions on an aspect of your care, for example. The project should be fully explained to you and you are free to decline, but your participation will be most welcome. Such projects are vital if professionals are to improve maternity care.

STUDENTS

Many of the professionals mentioned have students accompanying them at times. They will be at various stages of their training but will always be supervised. You can choose not to be seen by a student at any time but agreeing to their presence helps in their education and may even add to your experience of pregnancy and labour.

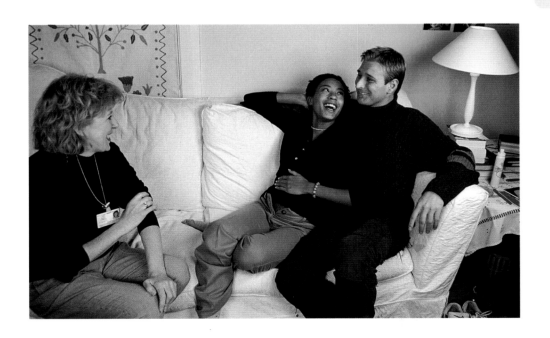

ANTENATAL CLASSES

Think about what you hope to gain from antenatal classes so that, if there is a choice, you can find the sort of class that suits you best. You need to start making enquiries early in pregnancy so that you can be sure of getting a place in the class you choose. You can go to more than one class. Ask your midwife, or health visitor, your GP, or the local branch of the National Childbirth Trust (see page 141).

'My midwife told me about a class specially for teenagers. It was great being with girls my age.'

'It really helped me to make up my mind about how I wanted to have my baby.'

Antenatal classes can help to prepare you for your baby's birth and for looking after and feeding your baby. They can also help you to keep yourself fit and well during pregnancy. They are often called parentcraft classes and may cover relaxation and breathing, and antenatal exercise. They're a good chance to meet other parents, to talk about things that might be worrying you and to ask questions – and to make new friends. They are usually informal and fun.

You may be able to go to some introductory classes on babycare early in pregnancy. Otherwise, many classes will start about eight to ten weeks before your baby is due. Classes are normally held once a week, either during the day or in the evening and last one or two hours. Some classes are for expectant women only. Others will welcome partners, either to all the sessions or to some of them, or you can go alone or with a friend. In some areas there are classes especially for women whose first language is not English, classes for single mothers and classes for teenagers. The kinds of topics covered by antenatal classes are:

- health in pregnancy;

- what happens during labour and birth;

- coping with labour and information about pain relief;

- exercises to keep you fit during pregnancy and help you in labour;

- relaxation;

- caring for your baby, including feeding;

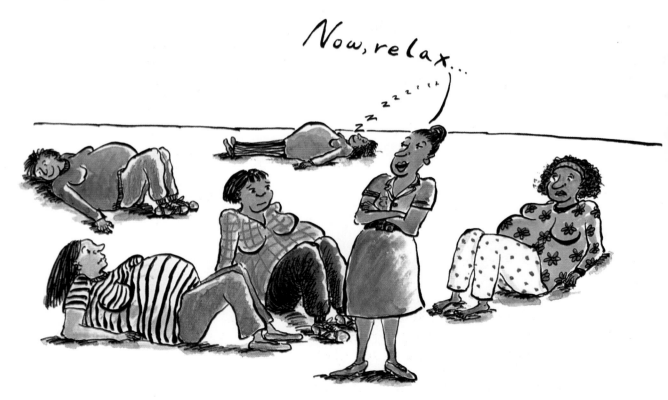

Now, relax...

64

- your own health after the birth;

- 'refresher classes' for those who have already had a baby;

- emotions surrounding pregnancy, birth and the early postnatal period.

Some classes will try to cover all these topics. Others will concentrate more on certain aspects, such as exercises and relaxation or babycare.

The number of different antenatal classes available varies very much from place to place. Classes may be run by your hospital, by your local midwives or health visitors, by your own GP or health centre. The National Childbirth Trust also runs classes, usually in the evenings and in the leader's home. The groups tend to be smaller and may go into more depth.

Antenatal classes may give you the opportunity to get to know some of the professionals involved in your care and to ask questions and talk over any worries you may have. You can find out about arrangements for labour and birth and the sort of choices available to you. This can help you in thinking about making your own birth plan (see page 38). You'll usually be able to look round the labour and postnatal wards. You may also be able to meet some of the people who will be looking after you when the time comes for your baby to be born.

Classes can give you confidence as well as information. You'll be able to talk over any worries and discuss your plans, not just with professionals, but with other parents as well.

Speak to your community midwife if you can't go to classes. The midwife may have videos to lend you or you may be able to hire or buy one.

'It was great meeting people who were going through the same things I was.'

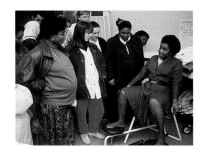

'It was brilliant having classes in the evening because it meant Phil could help me during labour.'

'Being shown the delivery suite helped us – just knowing what to expect made it less scary.'

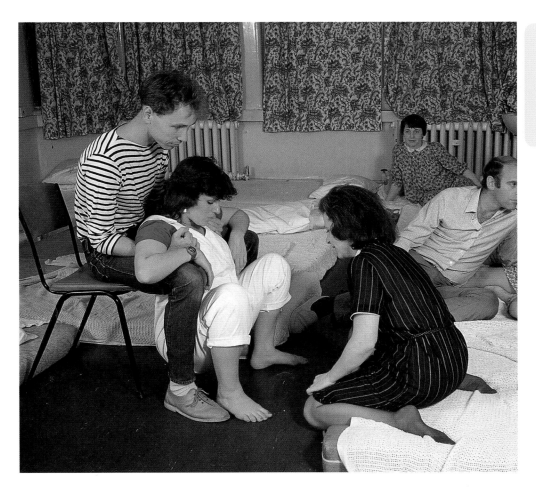

Classes may be available in your area for specific groups such as single women and teenagers. Ask your midwife for details.

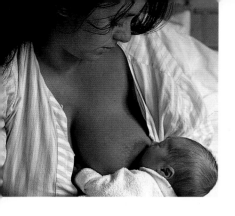

8 The feeding question

'It was so easy. I suppose it took me about a couple of weeks to get used to it, and from then on I just didn't have to think. It was the one thing that wasn't any effort at all.'

'Breastfeeding was so difficult what with one thing and another – first the baby was ill, then me. I'd be crying. The baby would be crying and hungry. So we started on the bottle and somehow from then on it was all right and I felt much better about it all.'

It's never too early to start thinking about how you're going to feed your baby. Once your baby is born there will be lots to occupy you! You'll need to discuss it with other people, the baby's father, your midwife, health visitor or other mothers.

Breastfeeding gives your baby the best possible start in life. Almost all women can breastfeed successfully though, as with all new skills, it may take some practice to get it right. If you have been told you cannot breastfeed or have tried but have not managed successfully, don't feel guilty about it. Accept the situation for what it is and enjoy the different benefits of bottle feeding. Even if you don't manage to breastfeed your first baby, it's still worth a go with your next baby – many women succeed the second time around.

If you decide not to breastfeed, it's important to know that it's very difficult to change from bottle to breastfeeding. If you like, you can breastfeed your baby for a year or more, but you may decide to breastfeed for a shorter time (if for example you are returning to work) and then change to bottle feeding. The following information should help you decide what's best for you and your baby.

If you're HIV positive you will be advised not to breastfeed because of the risk of passing the virus on to your baby through the milk. It is a good idea to discuss this with your midwife or doctor.

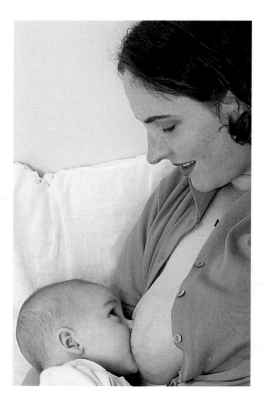

WATER

You may be advised to give your baby water between feeds if he or she cries, in case the baby is thirsty rather than hungry. This is not necessary. Even in very hot countries no extra water is needed. This is true for both breast and bottle-fed babies. Offer your baby a feed even if she or he has been fed recently. It is important to feed on demand since babies often don't conform to routine. This is particularly important for breastfed babies because they increase the milk supply by increasing the frequency of feeds. If your baby still won't settle, go through the checklist on page 119.

66

BREASTFEEDING

WHY BREAST IS BEST FOR BABIES

- Breast milk is the only food naturally designed for your baby. It contains the nutrients your baby needs in the right amounts and they are in a form that is very easily absorbed. Its composition even changes as your baby grows.

- Breastfeeding helps to protect your baby from infection because antibodies are passed into the milk. Your baby will be less vulnerable to coughs and colds and other infections than bottle-fed babies. If you breastfeed for the first three to four months, this protection can last for up to a year.

- Breast milk is easily digested and absorbed and is less likely to cause stomach upsets or diarrhoea. It will also help to avoid constipation in your baby.

- Breastfed babies are less likely to get allergies like eczema, for example.

- Breast milk contains growth factors and hormones to assist your baby's development.

WHY BREAST IS BEST FOR MOTHERS

As one mother said, 'It was feeling close, and being together, that was what I liked', but there are other benefits too.

- Breast milk costs nothing.

- There's no need to prepare feeds or wash and sterilise bottles.

- Your baby isn't kept waiting for a feed.

- Breastfeeding helps your womb return to its normal size more quickly and, because it uses up calories, it will help you to lose some of the weight gained in pregnancy.

- It's so much easier and more practical in the middle of the night.

'I didn't want to breastfeed. It was as simple as that. The whole idea of it put me off and I just couldn't have done it.'

'I had quite a few problems at first with sore nipples and one thing and another. It made it difficult. I think I'd have given up if it hadn't been for the midwife. She was ever so good. And after a while it all sorted out and now I'm glad I did it.'

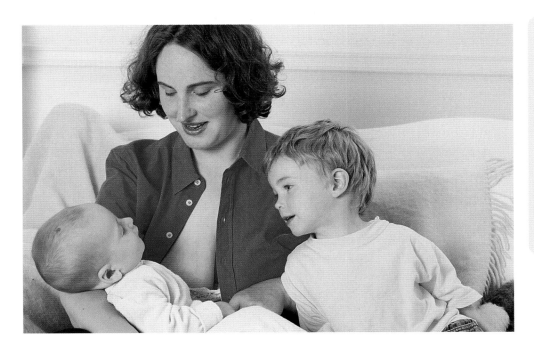

NURSING BRAS

A nursing bra will give you support so that you feel more comfortable. Ask for a proper fitting when choosing a bra. Choose adjustable bras because the size of your breasts will change (see page 88). Some women feel more comfortable wearing a nursing bra at night as well.

SOME OF YOUR QUESTIONS ANSWERED

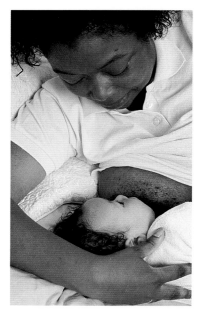

Can all women breastfeed?

Almost every woman can breastfeed, but it can sometimes take a little while to get it right. Be patient and ask your midwife or health visitor for help if you need it.

Does breast size matter?

No. All shapes and sizes make milk.

Can flat or inverted nipples be a problem?

Most women with flat or inverted nipples should be able to breastfeed. However, you may need a little extra help in learning to position your baby (see page 70).

Do I need to prepare my breasts for breastfeeding?

Your breasts will prepare themselves naturally, although it's a good idea to try to keep your skin soft and supple, so avoid soaps and sprays that have a drying effect.

If my baby is born prematurely, will it have the energy to suck at the breast?

Maybe not at first, but small babies will benefit if they get some mother's milk as it is exactly right for them. You can express your milk and you can give it by bottle, tube or cup, if your baby can't take it directly from your breast.

How can I make sure my partner feels involved?

Breastfeeding is only one way to be close to a baby. Your partner can cuddle and bathe the baby and perhaps give bottles of expressed milk later on.

Can I go out without the baby?

Yes, you can express some of your milk and leave it for someone else to give your baby (see page 72).

Is it worth breastfeeding if I am going back to work soon?

Yes. The early weeks, while you are at home, are the time when breast milk does the most good. After that you can express your breast milk or use infant formula milk for your baby while you are at work and continue to breastfeed at other times.

What about feeding my baby in front of friends or in public?

You may be quite happy about feeding in front of others. If you feel uneasy, you could feed the baby discreetly under a loose top, T-shirt or half-unbuttoned blouse. Don't be embarrassed to ask if there's a mother and baby room when you're out.

Should I give my baby any other drinks?

Breastfed babies do not need any other drinks, including infant fruit juices, herb teas or boiled water, providing you feed them whenever they ask. You yourself may be more thirsty during breastfeeding, so be sure to drink plenty of fluids.

How long should I breastfeed for?

You can go on as long as you want to. Breastfeeding for at least the first four months gives your baby the best start in life. If you can, continue to give some breastfeeds until your baby's first birthday. After that, he or she can have whole cow's milk as a drink. If you switch to formula feeds you can still breastfeed your baby once or twice a day. This way your baby will continue to benefit from your breast milk.

Breastfeeding a baby can be a great pleasure. Even if it doesn't go well for you at the start, it's still worth working at. Although problems with breastfeeding, even fairly small problems, can be quite upsetting, they can almost always be overcome.

'I didn't realise that bottle feeding would be so much trouble. It was really hard to find time to sterilise and make up the bottles. My new baby took up all my time.'

'I really enjoy the closeness of breastfeeding and my partner says it makes him feel so proud, watching us together.'

You can get help from:

- your midwife or health visitor;

- a breastfeeding counsellor or support group (contact your local branch of the National Childbirth Trust, or the La Lèche League (page 141 – these organisations give help and support through other mothers who have experience of breastfeeding).

Don't worry if other mothers seem to be doing things differently. It is important to have confidence in yourself and your baby so that together you can work out what is best for both of you.

THE FIRST FEW DAYS

In the beginning, it can seem that you are doing nothing but feeding, but gradually your baby will settle into a pattern of feeding. Try to relax into it and take each day as it comes.

For the first few days after birth your breasts produce a special food called **colostrum**, which looks like rich creamy milk and is sometimes quite yellow in colour. This contains all the food your baby needs, as well as antibodies which pass your own resistance to certain infections on to your baby.

After about three days your breasts will begin to produce milk which will look quite thin compared with colostrum. The milk now varies according to the needs of your baby. The **fore milk**, which your baby takes first, is thirst-quenching and means your baby gets a drink at the start of every feed. A breastfed baby doesn't need any other drinks (including infant teas or juices), even in hot weather, as long as you feed whenever the baby asks. The fore milk is then followed by the richer **hind milk**.

This is the food part of the feed and contains the calories your baby needs. This is why you shouldn't restrict the length of feeds or swap breasts after too short a time. Your breasts may become very large and heavy for a while and may feel uncomfortable, or even painful, at first.

Milk may leak from your nipples and you may feel more comfortable wearing breast pads. Change them frequently. Avoid plastic backs. Or you can use clean cotton hankies, and at night you could put a clean towel under you instead of wearing pads.

Gradually the amount of milk you produce will settle down and your breasts will begin to feel normal again. If you are very uncomfortable, ask your midwife, health visitor or breastfeeding counsellor for help.

HOW BREASTFEEDING WORKS

Your milk supply
Your breasts produce milk in response to your baby feeding at your breast. The more your baby feeds, the more your body makes milk, provided that your baby is correctly positioned. If you reduce feeding, you will make less milk.

The 'let-down' reflex
Your baby's sucking causes milk to gather behind the nipple, ready for feeding. This is called the 'let-down' reflex; some mothers feel it as a tingling sensation. You will see quick sucks change to deep swallows once the milk has begun to flow. Babies often pause while they wait for more milk to be 'delivered'. Anxiety or tiredness can stop the 'let-down' reflex, so try to rest and relax as much as you can while you are breastfeeding.

A supplement of vitamins A, C and D, plus seven pints of cow's milk per week are available free to pregnant and breastfeeding mothers if your family receives Income Support or Jobseeker's Allowance. Use the free milk as a drink, on cereals or to make sauces and puddings. The vitamin drops are available to all mothers at very low cost. Ask your midwife or health visitor about it.

'I wasn't sure if I'd be able to breastfeed. My mum bottle fed me so she couldn't help. Once I got going though, it was so easy. I can't think now why I was so unsure at first.'

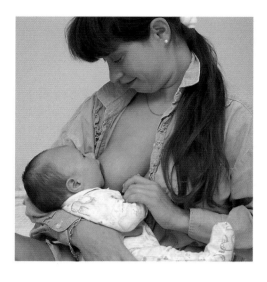

IMPORTANT POINTS TO REMEMBER

- *If your baby just feeds on the nipple, he or she will get very little milk and you may become sore.*

- *If feeding feels wrong or hurts or your baby doesn't seem to be feeding properly, stop the feed. Break the suction by putting your little finger into the corner of your baby's mouth. Adjust the position and start again.*

- *Breastfeeding may be a little uncomfortable at first as your nipples may be sore, but this will soon ease, providing your baby is correctly positioned on the breast, as you and your baby become accustomed to this new skill.*

HOW TO BREASTFEED

As with all new skills, you'll need a little practice – ask your midwife to show you what to do. Your midwife, health visitor or breastfeeding counsellor will be pleased to help. The following hints will give you a few basic ideas.

- First find a comfortable position, either sitting upright, well supported or lying down. Cushions or pillows may help to support you and your baby.

- Then turn your baby towards you with the head and shoulders opposite your breast and the nose opposite your nipple. Support your baby with a hand across the shoulders, not behind the head.

- Now brush your baby's lips against your nipple to get his or her mouth open really wide, then draw your baby to your breast quickly. If you gently stroke down your breast towards the nipple to express a little milk, your baby may find it easier to latch on. If your baby is correctly positioned, there will be more of your areola (the brown skin around the nipple) showing above the top lip than below the bottom lip.

- Start each feed on alternate breasts. Let your baby decide when he or she has finished the first breast before switching to the second. Sometimes babies only need one breast at a feed.

- Many babies will develop a pattern of feeding. You should feed your baby on demand and not let the baby wait for a feed or restrict the length of feeds.

HOW OFTEN AND HOW MUCH

It's best to feed when your baby wants to be fed. This might be very often at first, though feeds will become more spaced out as your baby gets older. Some babies settle

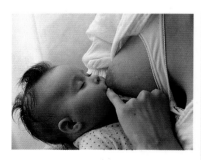

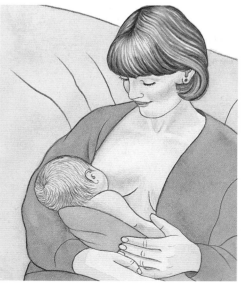

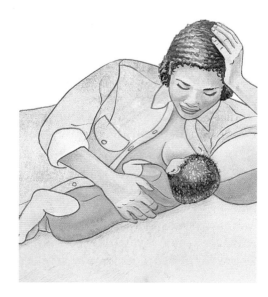

into their own pattern quite quickly, others take longer.

From time to time, your baby will have a growth spurt – usually around 10 days, 6 weeks and 12 weeks. When this happens, your baby needs more milk and you may find that feeds are longer and more frequent. Don't panic and feel you need to offer extra bottles of infant formula milk. You'll make more milk in response to your baby's demands, but this may take a day or two, so be patient. The frequency and length of feeds will then settle.

The sucking process releases milk to satisfy your baby and stimulates the production of more. When your baby is full up, he or she will stop feeding. Plenty of wet nappies is a good sign that your baby is getting enough fluid. If you're worried, talk to your midwife, health visitor or breastfeeding counsellor.

HOW TO OVERCOME COMMON DIFFICULTIES

The quicker you sort out any difficulties in breastfeeding, the better for you and your baby. So don't hesitate to ask for help immediately. Many women are surprised to find that most problems are quite easily overcome by a slight change to their baby's position when feeding or by feeding their baby more often.

Feeding restlessly
If your baby is restless at the breast and doesn't seem satisfied by feeds, it may be that he or she is sucking on the nipple alone and so not getting enough milk. Ask for help in making sure your baby feeds in the right position.

Engorged breasts
A few days after the birth, your breasts may become very swollen (engorged) and uncomfortable. The

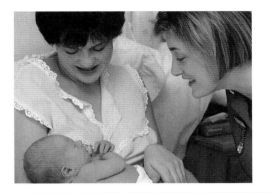

YOUR DIET WHEN BREASTFEEDING

Try to eat well at meal times, with plenty of pasta, potatoes, bread and rice, and have healthy snacks in between (see page 11). Drink plenty of fluids, especially in hot weather and keep your intake of alcohol low. Don't go on a crash course to lose weight. Your milk will be affected and you will probably feel more tired. Breastfeeding and healthy eating should help you to lose any surplus pounds naturally and gradually.

It can be difficult to make sure you get enough vitamin D; it is present in only a few foods, such as fortified margarines, oily fish, eggs and milk. But it's also made by the skin when it is exposed to 'gentle' summer sunlight (remember to apply a high-factor sunscreen). If you're not sure you're getting enough, especially during the winter months, you may need to take vitamin D supplement. They're available cheaply from health centres, and they're free of charge if your family receives Income Support or Jobseeker's Allowance. Always talk to your doctor or health visitor before taking supplements.

SHOULD I AVOID ANYTHING?

*Breastfeeding should be an enjoyable time for you and your baby. There should be no need to avoid eating any foods, but if you, your baby's father or any previous children have a history of hayfever, asthma, eczema or other allergies, avoid eating peanuts and foods containing peanut products (e.g. peanut butter, **unrefined** groundnut oils and some snacks, etc.). This may reduce the risk of your baby developing a potentially serious allergy to peanuts. Read food labels carefully and if you are still in doubt about the contents these foods should be avoided. Some mothers say that certain foods they eat (e.g. onions, garlic, citrus fruits and grapes) seem to upset their baby. However, it's important to check with a health professional before you omit foods from your diet because it is possible to become deficient in certain minerals or vitamins by doing this.*

Small amounts of alcohol pass into the breast milk, making it smell different to your baby, and may affect his or her feeding, sleeping or digestion. So keep within the daily benchmark for women of between 2–3 units or less a day (see page 14). Medicines (prescribed or over the counter) may also pass into breast milk, so check first with your GP to be quite sure. Always tell your doctor, dentist or pharmacist that you are breastfeeding.

*'Knowing that my baby was growing and putting on weight because of milk from **me** made me feel really proud.'*

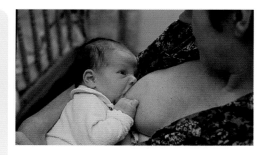

answer is to breastfeed. If feeding is difficult for any reason, ask your midwife for help or make sure you have the telephone number of a breastfeeding counsellor. A good supporting bra will help too, but make sure it isn't too tight.

Sore or cracked nipples

If your nipples are sore when you're feeding, your baby's position may need adjusting. If they are cracked, get advice from your midwife, health visitor or GP as cracked nipples can lead to breast infection. The following suggestions may also help:

- keep your nipples dry and expose them to the air as much as you can — try sleeping topless if it's warm enough, with a towel under you if you're leaking milk;

- change your breast pads frequently (use pads without plastic);

- avoid soap as it dries the skin;

- wear a cotton bra which allows air to circulate;

- try squeezing out a drop or two of your milk at the end of a feed and gently rubbing it into your skin.

If you suddenly get sore and pink nipples after any first soreness has passed, you might have an infection known as thrush. Go and see your GP.

Lumpy tender breasts

This can happen if a milk duct becomes blocked. Milk builds up because the ducts aren't being emptied. There are a number of things you can do to help:

- let your baby feed on the tender breast first or, if he or she doesn't want to feed, try expressing some milk;

- while your baby is feeding, gently stroke the lumpy area with your fingertips, smoothing the milk towards your nipple;

- try leaning over your baby as you feed.

It's important to deal with a blocked duct as soon as possible to make sure that it doesn't lead to mastitis (infection in your breast).

Mastitis

If you have mastitis your breasts will feel hot and tender and you may feel as though you have flu. If this occurs, continue to breastfeed but get a midwife or health visitor to check your position. Try the suggestions above for lumpy, tender breasts and get lots of rest. Go to bed if you can. See your GP if there is no improvement within six to eight hours as you may need antibiotics to clear the infection. Your doctor can prescribe one which is safe to take whilst breastfeeding.

WIND

Babies may take in air as they feed — bottle-fed babies more than breastfed babies. After a feed, gentle back rubbing with your baby lying against your shoulder or held a little forward on your lap may bring up some wind that would be uncomfortable otherwise. Don't worry if you don't get any up. It is not essential. It may even be that there is none to come. Sometimes a little milk is brought up at the same time. This is known as **posset** and it's normal.

BOTTLE FEEDING

Bottle feeding may seem like hard work at first until you get into a routine of sterilising bottles and preparing feeds. Once you're organised, you'll be able to relax and really enjoy feeding. Feeding is the best time to hold your baby close in your arms and one advantage of bottle feeding is that fathers can share in this enjoyment.

BABY MILK (INFANT FORMULA)

Baby milk, also called infant formula or artificial milk, usually comes in powder form. It is usually cow's milk that has been specially treated so that babies can digest it. And it has the right balance of vitamins and minerals for a young baby. Baby milks based on soya protein are also available but they are not usually given at this young age.

Ordinary cow's milk, condensed milk, evaporated milk, dried milk, goat's milk, or any other type of milk should never be given to a baby. They are not suitable. If you have any worries about the baby milk you are giving your baby, ask advice from your midwife, health visitor or GP.

There are a number of different brands of baby milk available in the shops. 'Ready-to-feed' baby milks in cartons are also available in some places. This is generally more expensive than powdered milk but may be useful in an emergency or if you're away from home. Once opened, the carton should be stored in the fridge and thrown away after 24 hours.

Although formula milk contains vitamins, you may be advised to give your baby vitamin drops from the age of six months onwards, or earlier in some special cases. You can buy these at the Child Health Clinic or any pharmacy.

SOYA-BASED INFANT FORMULAE

If you have chosen to bottle feed but your baby cannot tolerate cow's milk formula, your GP or health visitor may have advised that you feed your baby with a formula based on soya. These formulae are made wholly from plants and so vegan parents may prefer to use them instead of cow's milk formulae. Remember though that breast milk is the best food for your baby.

There has recently been some concern over phytoestrogens, a **natural** component of the soya bean. There is no evidence at present that feeding your baby with soya-based formulae will cause any problems, but research is being undertaken to give a better understanding of the effects phytoestrogens have on the body. If you are using soya-based formulae because of cow's milk intolerance, remember that babies can grow out of allergies so it may be possible to introduce cow's milk into your baby's diet as he or she gets older. Do not make any changes to your baby's diet without first seeking advice from your GP or health visitor.

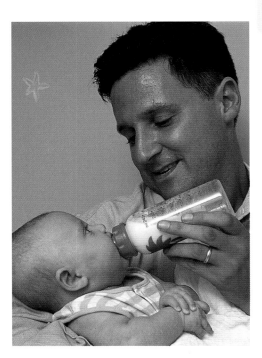

'Because Ellen was bottle-fed we both fed her. I used to do it in the evenings and most of the feeds at weekends. We started to do it to give Karen a rest, but in the end I wanted to do it. It brought the baby closer. She's very close to me now.'

(A FATHER)

'When I saw women breastfeeding at my postnatal group, I felt that we'd missed out by using bottles. I'll give breastfeeding a try next time.'

If you are bottle feeding and you're on Income Support or income-based Jobseeker's Allowance you can get tokens for free milk and vitamins for your baby (see page 133). Vitamins may be recommended from six months or earlier in some cases.

Feeding is a time for getting to know your baby and feeling close. But remember, even when your baby is a little older, he or she should never be left alone to feed with a propped-up bottle in case of choking.

USING BOTTLED WATER

If you use bottled water to make up a feed, for example on holiday, it must be boiled and then cooled first. Use spring water not mineral water. Use still water, not fizzy.

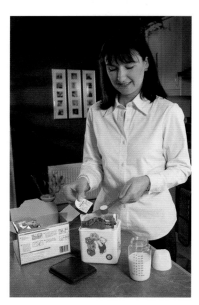

BOTTLES AND TEATS

You'll need at least six bottles and teats. This is to make sure that you always have at least one or two bottles clean, sterilised and ready for use. Ask your midwife, health visitor or other mothers if you want advice on what kind to buy.

You should always buy new teats and it's best if you can buy new bottles too. Check regularly to make sure the bottles are in good condition. If they're badly scratched, you won't be able to sterilise them properly. If in doubt, ask your midwife or health visitor for advice.

MAKING UP THE FEED

When you're preparing formula milk, always **follow the instructions on the tin exactly**. Remember to put the boiled water into the bottle first. The milk powder has been very carefully balanced for your baby, so don't be tempted to add extra powder to make a 'stronger feed' as this could be harmful to your baby. Never use less or more than instructed and don't add any other ingredients such as sugar, honey, rusks or baby rice.

If you're worried, your midwife or health visitor will advise you how much milk your baby is likely to need. If you make up more than your baby wants, throw away what is left at the end of the feed. You will probably find it suits your routine to make up a number of feeds in advance. Cool the capped bottles quickly under cold running water and put them in the fridge as soon as possible. Don't keep the made up milk for longer than 24 hours.

FEEDING

Your baby will gradually settle into a routine. Babies vary in how often they want to feed and how much they want to take. Some may be content with feeds every three to four hours and others may want smaller quantities more often. Respond to your baby's needs and feed when he or she is hungry, just as you would if you were breastfeeding. In the same way, don't try to force your baby to finish a bottle. He or she may have had enough for the time being or simply want a rest.

The temperature of the milk
Before you start to feed your baby always check that the milk is not too hot by dripping some on the inside of your wrist. Some babies don't mind cold milk. Others prefer it warm. If you want to warm the milk a little, place the bottle upright in some hot water, keeping the teat out of the water. Don't keep the milk warm for more than 20 minutes before the feed as germs can breed in the warmth. Never warm the milk in a microwave oven as this is unsafe. The milk continues to heat for a time after you take it out of the microwave, even though the outside of the bottle may feel cold. The milk inside may be very hot and could scald your baby's mouth.

A comfortable position
Have everything you need ready before you start feeding.

Find a comfortable position in which you can hold your baby while you are feeding. Give your baby time. Some babies take some milk, pause for a nap and then wake up for more. So be patient.

The teat

As you feed, keep the bottle tilted so that the teat is always full of milk. Otherwise your baby will be taking in air. If the teat becomes flattened while you are feeding pull gently on the bottle to release the vacuum. If the teat becomes blocked, replace it with another sterile teat. Teats do come in different shapes and with different hole sizes. You may have to try several before you find the one that suits your baby. If the hole is too small your baby will not get enough milk. If it's too big it will come too fast. Check that the teat is not torn or damaged.

After the feed

Gently rub or pat your baby's back for a while to see whether there is any wind to come up. There's no need to overdo this. Wind is not such a problem as many people think. But your baby will probably enjoy the rubbing and closeness to you after the feed.

Don't forget to throw away unused milk in the bottle.

Your midwife or health visitor will chat to you about feeding when they call at your home or you could telephone them or see them at your Child Health Clinic. Talk to them about any worries or problems you may have.

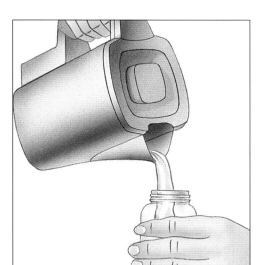

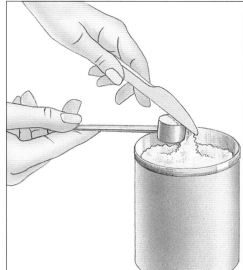

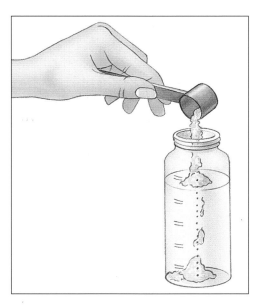

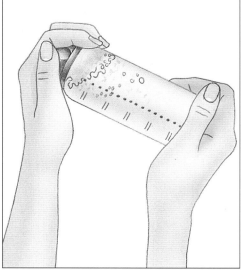

PREPARING A FEED

1 *Make sure your hands are absolutely clean.*

2 *Boil some water in the kettle and let it cool.*

3 *Take a sterilised bottle and teat.*

4 *Take the cooled water and fill the bottle to the right place using the measuring marks.*

5 *Measure the exact amount of powder using the special scoop provided with the milk. Level off the powder in the scoop using a clean dry knife. Don't pack the powder down at all.*

6 *Add the powder to the water in the bottle.*

7 *Screw on the cap and shake well until the powder has dissolved.*

8 *Store the bottle in the fridge if you're not using it straight away.*

CLEANING AND STERILISING

It's important to keep bottles and teats, and other equipment used in feeding, absolutely clean to protect your baby against infection. This means sterilising as well as washing. There are a number of different ways to do this. You can use:

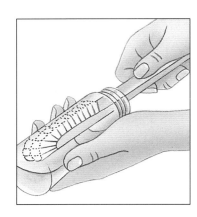

- **a chemical steriliser** – there are several different brands in the shops, and consist of a sterilising tank to which you add cold water and a sterilising tablet or liquid;

- **a steam steriliser** – this is a very quick and efficient method of sterilising;

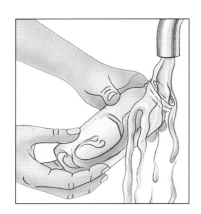

- **a microwave bottle steriliser** – a microwave alone is not enough to sterilise the bottles without this equipment.

Ask your midwife, health visitor or other mothers about the different methods and which might be most appropriate for you. If you buy equipment, make sure you follow the manufacturer's instructions.

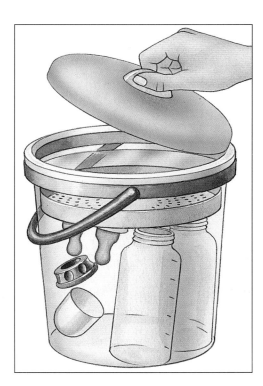

Chemical sterilisation

1 Wash the bottles, teats and other equipment thoroughly in hot water using washing-up liquid. Get rid of every trace of milk using a bottle brush for the inside of the bottles. You may have been advised to use salt to clean the teats, but this is no longer recommended. Squirt water through the teats. This will make sure the holes are clear.

2 Rinse thoroughly in clean running water.

3 To make up the solution, follow the instructions that come with the sterilising tablets or liquid. Put the bottles and teats and other equipment (but nothing metal) in the solution and leave for the time given in the instructions. The tank will have a floating lid that keeps everything under the water or you can use a large plate to keep the bottles immersed. Make sure there are no air bubbles inside the bottles. Put the teats and caps in upside down to prevent air being trapped. Once the equipment is sterilised you should not add new items or the whole solution will be contaminated.

4 Make sure your hands are absolutely clean when you take out the bottles and teats to make up the feeds. When you take out the bottles, shake off the water. It is not necessary to rinse the bottles but, if you do, use cooled boiled water. Do not use tap water as this will make them unsterile again.

9 Problems

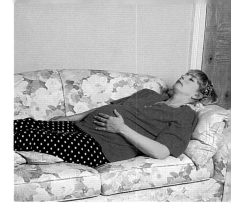

Your body has a great deal to do during pregnancy. Sometimes the changes taking place will cause irritation or discomfort, and on occasions they may seem quite alarming. There is rarely any need for alarm but you should mention anything that is worrying you to your doctor or midwife.

If you think that something may be seriously wrong, trust your own judgement and get in touch with your doctor or midwife straight away.

We have listed, in alphabetical order, the changes you are most likely to notice and their causes – where these are known – plus suggestions on how to cope.

COMMON MINOR PROBLEMS

BACKACHE

During pregnancy ligaments become softer and stretch to prepare you for labour. This can put a strain on the joints of your lower back and pelvis which can cause backache. As the baby grows, the hollow in your lower back may increase and this may also cause backache.

To avoid backache:

- avoid heavy lifting;

- bend your knees and keep your back straight when lifting or picking something up from the floor;

- if you do have to carry something heavy, hold it close to your body;

- move your feet when turning round to avoid twisting your spine;

- wear flat shoes as these allow your weight to be evenly distributed;

- work at a surface high enough to prevent you stooping;

- try to balance the weight between two baskets if you are carrying shopping;

- sit with your back straight and well supported.

A firm mattress can help to prevent and relieve backache. If your mattress is too soft, a piece of hardboard under its length will make it firmer.

Massage can also help, or you might like to try a support corset – these can be prescribed by the doctor. Make sure you get enough rest, particularly later in pregnancy.

If your backache is very painful, ask your doctor to refer you to an obstetric physiotherapist at your hospital. He or she will be able to give you some advice and suggest some helpful exercises.

CONSTIPATION

You may become constipated very early in pregnancy because of the hormonal changes going on in your body. It will help to:

- make sure you include plenty of fibre in your diet through eating foods like wholemeal breads, wholegrain cereals, fruit and vegetables, and pulses such as beans and lentils;

- exercise regularly to keep your muscles toned up;

- make sure you drink plenty of water;

- avoid iron pills if they cause constipation – ask your doctor whether you can manage without them or change to a different type; if not, you may have to accept having constipation.

CRAMP

Cramp is a sudden, sharp pain, usually in your calf muscles or feet. It is most common at night, but nobody really knows what causes it. It usually helps if you pull your toes hard up towards your ankle or rub the muscle hard. Regular, gentle exercise in pregnancy, particularly ankle and leg movements, will improve your circulation and may help to prevent cramp occurring.

DISCHARGE FROM BREASTS

You may notice a discharge from your nipples. This is very common and nothing to worry about. However, see your doctor or midwife if it becomes bloodstained.

FAINTNESS

Pregnant women often feel faint. This happens when not enough blood is getting to the brain. If the oxygen level gets too low you may actually faint. It's more common in pregnancy because of hormonal changes taking place in your body. You're most likely to feel faint if you stand still for too long or get up too quickly from a chair or hot bath. It often happens when you are lying on your back.

- Try to get up slowly after sitting or lying down.

- If you feel faint when standing still, find a seat quickly and the faintness will pass. If it doesn't, lie down on your side.

- If you feel faint while lying on your back, turn on to your side. It's better not to lie flat on your back in later pregnancy or during labour.

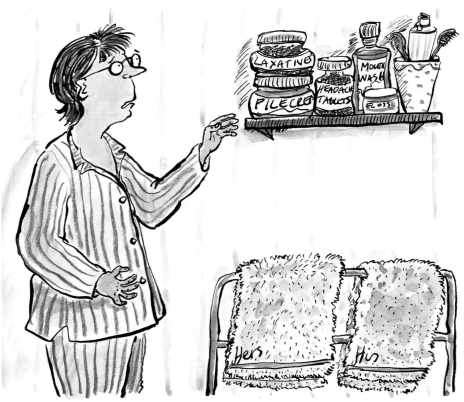

FEELING HOT IN PREGNANCY

During pregnancy you're likely to feel warmer than normal. This is due to hormonal changes and to an increase in blood supply to the skin. You're also likely to sweat more. It helps if you:

- wear loose clothing made of natural fibres, as these are more absorbent and 'breathe' more than synthetic fibres;

- keep your room cool – consider using an electric fan;

- wash frequently to stay fresh.

HEADACHES

Some pregnant women find they get a lot of headaches. A brisk walk may be all you need, as well as a little more regular rest and relaxation. Although it is wise to avoid drugs in pregnancy, an occasional paracetamol tablet is generally considered safe.

If you often have bad headaches, tell your doctor or midwife so that they can advise you. Severe headaches may be a sign of high blood pressure (see page 84).

INDIGESTION AND HEARTBURN

This is partly caused by hormonal changes and later the growing womb pressing on the stomach. If you suffer from indigestion:

- try eating smaller meals more often;

- sit up straight when you are eating as this takes the pressure off your stomach;

- avoid particular foods which cause trouble, for example fried

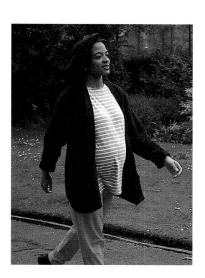

or highly spiced ones, but make sure you are still eating well (see pages 8-12 for information on healthy eating).

Heartburn is more than just indigestion. It is a strong, burning pain in the chest. It is caused by the valve between your stomach and the tube leading to your stomach relaxing in pregnancy, so that stomach acid passes into the tube. It is often brought on by lying flat. To avoid heartburn you could:

- sleep well propped up – try raising the head of your bed with bricks or have plenty of pillows;

- try drinking a glass of milk – have one by your bed in case you wake with heartburn in the night;

- avoiding eating or drinking for a few hours before you go to bed;

- ask your doctor or midwife for advice;

- don't take antacid tablets or mixture before checking that they are safe in pregnancy.

ITCHING

Mild itching is common in pregnancy because of the increased blood supply to the skin. In late pregnancy the skin of the abdomen is stretched and this may also cause itchiness. Wearing loose clothing may help.

Itching can, however, be a sign of a more serious problem called obstetric cholestasis (see page 84). If itching becomes severe, or you develop jaundice (yellowing of the whites of the eyes and skin), see your doctor. Itching which is associated with a rash may also need treatment if it is severe.

NAUSEA AND MORNING SICKNESS

Nausea is very common in the early weeks of pregnancy. Some women feel sick, some are sick. Some feel sick in the mornings, some at other times, some all day long.

The reasons are not fully understood, but hormonal changes in the first three months are probably one cause. Nausea usually disappears around the 12th to 14th week. Nausea can be one of the most trying problems in early pregnancy. It comes at a time when you may be feeling tired and emotional, and when many people around you may not realise you are pregnant and expect you to be your normal self.

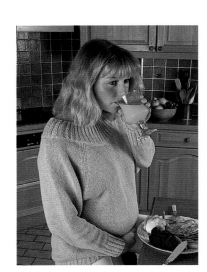

- If you feel sick first thing in the morning, give yourself time to get up slowly. If possible, eat something like dry toast or a plain biscuit before you get up. Your partner could bring you some sweet tea.

- Get plenty of rest and sleep whenever you can. Feeling tired can make the sickness worse.

- Eat small amounts often rather than several large meals, but don't stop eating.

- Drink plenty of fluids.

- Ask those close to you for extra support.

- Distract yourself as much as you can. Often the nausea gets worse the more you think about it.

- Avoid the foods and smells that make you feel worse. It helps if someone else can cook but, if not, go for bland, non-greasy foods such as baked potatoes, pasta and milk puddings, which are simple to prepare.

- Remedies containing ginger may be helpful.

- Wear comfortable clothes. Tight waistbands can make you feel worse.

If you can't keep anything down see your doctor or midwife.

NOSE BLEEDS

Nose bleeds are quite common in pregnancy because of hormonal changes. The nose bleeds are usually short but can be quite heavy. To help the bleeding stop, press the sides of your nose together between your thumb and forefinger just below the bony part of your nose for ten minutes. Repeat for a further ten minutes if this is unsuccessful. As long as you don't lose a lot of blood, there is nothing to worry about. Blow your nose gently and try to avoid explosive sneezes. You may also find that your nose gets more blocked up than usual.

PASSING WATER OFTEN

Needing to pass water often is an early sign of pregnancy. Sometimes it continues right through pregnancy. In later pregnancy it's the result of the baby's head pressing on the bladder.

If you find that you're having to get up in the night, you could try cutting out drinks in the late evening but make sure you keep drinking plenty during the day. Later in pregnancy, some women find it helps to rock backwards and forwards while they are on the toilet. This lessens the pressure of the womb on the bladder so that you can empty it properly. Then you won't need to pass water again quite so soon.

If you have any pain while passing water, or pass any blood, you may have a urine infection which will need treatment. Drink plenty of water to dilute your urine and reduce irritation. You should contact your GP within 24 hours.

Sometimes pregnant women are unable to prevent a sudden spurt of urine or a small leak when they cough, sneeze or laugh, or when moving suddenly or just getting up from a sitting position. This may be temporary because the pelvic floor muscles relax slightly to prepare for the baby's delivery.

The growing baby will increase pressure on the bladder. If you find this a problem, you can improve the situation by doing exercises to tone up your pelvic floor muscles (see page 16). Ask a midwife or obstetric physiotherapist (see pages 62 and 63) for advice.

PILES

Piles, also known as haemorrhoids, are swollen veins around the back passage which may itch, ache or feel sore. You can usually feel the lumpiness of the piles around the back passage. Piles may also bleed a little and they can make going to the toilet uncomfortable or even painful. They occur in pregnancy because the veins relax under the influence of pregnancy hormones. Piles usually go shortly after delivery. If you suffer from piles you should:

- eat plenty of food that is high in fibre, like wholemeal bread, fruit and vegetables, and you should drink plenty of water – this will prevent constipation, which can make piles worse;

- avoid standing for long periods;

- take regular exercise to improve your circulation;

- sleep with the foot of the bed slightly raised on books or bricks;

- use an ice pack to ease discomfort, holding this gently against the piles, or use a cloth wrung out in iced water;

- if the piles stick out, push them gently back inside using a lubricating jelly;

- ask your doctor, midwife or pharmacist if they can suggest a suitable ointment;

- consider giving birth in a position where the pressure on your back passage is reduced – kneeling, for example.

SKIN AND HAIR CHANGES

Hormonal changes taking place in pregnancy will make your nipples and the area around them go darker. Your skin colour may also darken a little, either in patches or all over. Birthmarks, moles and freckles may also darken. Some women develop a dark line running down the middle of their stomachs. These changes will gradually fade after the baby has been born, although your nipples may remain a little darker.

If you sunbathe while you are pregnant, you may find you tan more easily. Protect your skin with a good, high-factor sunscreen. Don't stay in the sun for very long.

Hair growth is also likely to increase in pregnancy. Your hair may also be greasier. After the baby is born it may seem as if you're losing a lot of hair. In fact, you're simply losing the increase that occurred during pregnancy.

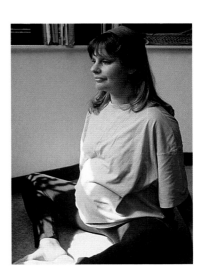

If you sometimes can't help wetting or soiling yourself, you can get help. Incontinence is a very common problem. It can affect anyone, sometimes during and after pregnancy. In many cases it is curable, so if you've got a problem talk to your doctor, midwife or health visitor, or ring the confidential Continence Foundation on (020) 7831 9831 (9.30–4.30 Mon–Fri).

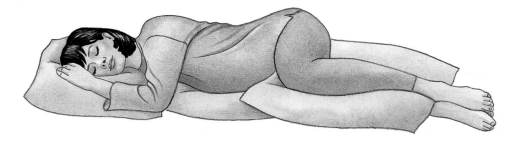

It might be more comfortable to lie on one side with a pillow under your tummy and another between your knees.

SLEEPLESSNESS

Late in pregnancy it can be very difficult to get a good night's sleep. You're uncomfortable lying down, or just when you're beginning to get comfortable you have to get up to go to the toilet. Some women have strange dreams or nightmares about the baby and about the birth. Talking about them can help you. Just because you dream something, it doesn't mean it's going to happen. Relaxation and breathing which are taught in antenatal classes might be helpful.

STRETCH MARKS

These are pink or purplish lines which usually occur on the tummy or sometimes on the upper thighs or breasts. Some women get them, some don't. It depends on your skin type. Some people's skin is more elastic. You are more likely to get stretch marks if your weight gain is more than average.

It's very doubtful whether oils or creams help to prevent stretch marks. After your baby is born the marks should gradually pale and become less noticeable.

SWOLLEN ANKLES, FEET AND FINGERS

Ankles, feet and fingers often swell a little in pregnancy because the body holds more water than usual. Towards the end of the day, especially if the weather is hot or if you have been standing a lot, the extra water tends

to gather in the lowest parts of the body. You should:

● try to avoid standing for long periods;

● wear comfortable shoes;

● put your feet up as much as you can – try to rest for an hour a day with your feet higher than your heart;

● try to do your foot exercises (see page 17) – these will help.

TEETH AND GUMS

Bleeding gums are caused by a build-up of plaque (bacteria) on the teeth. During pregnancy, hormonal changes in your body can cause the plaque to make the gums more inflamed. They may become swollen and bleed more easily. To keep your teeth and gums healthy, you should:

● pay special attention to cleaning your teeth. Ask your dentist to show you a good brushing method to remove all the plaque;

● avoid having sugary drinks and foods too often. Try to keep them only to meal times;

● remember that dental treatment is free while you are pregnant and for a year after your baby's birth, so have a check-up now;

● discuss with your dentist whether any new or replacement fillings should be delayed until after your baby is born.

Vaginal discharge

Almost all women have more vaginal discharge in pregnancy. It should be clear and white and it should not smell unpleasant. If the discharge is coloured or smells strange or if you feel itchy or sore, you may have a vaginal infection. Tell your doctor or midwife. The most common infection is thrush which your doctor can treat easily. You can help prevent thrush by wearing loose cotton underwear.

If vaginal discharge, of any colour, increases a lot in later pregnancy, tell your doctor or midwife.

Varicose veins

Varicose veins are veins which have become swollen. The veins in the legs are most commonly affected. You can also get varicose veins in the vulva (vaginal opening). They usually get better after delivery. You should:

- try to avoid standing for long periods of time;

- try not to sit with your legs crossed;

- try not to put on too much weight as this increases the pressure;

- sit with your legs up as often as you can to ease the discomfort;

- try support tights which may also help support the muscles of your legs – you can buy them at most pharmacists;

- try sleeping with your legs higher than the rest of your body – use pillows under your ankles or put bricks or books under the foot of your bed;

- do foot exercises (see page 17) and other antenatal exercises which will all help your circulation, such as walking, cycling, and swimming.

Tiredness

In the early months of pregnancy you may feel tired or even desperately exhausted. The only answer is to try to rest as much as possible. Make time to sit with your feet up during the day and accept any offers of help from colleagues and family. Towards the end of pregnancy, you may feel tired because of the extra weight you are carrying. Make sure you get plenty of rest.

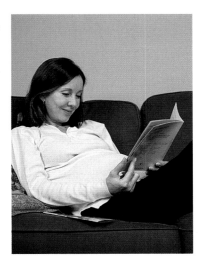

More serious problems

Slow-growing babies

Many of the tests in pregnancy check the growth of your baby. If you have previously had a very small baby, or if you smoke heavily, the midwives and doctors will already be monitoring your pregnancy closely. Blood pressure checks may also pick up signs of trouble. If there is concern about your baby's health, further tests may be carried out and more frequent monitoring of your baby may be recommended.

In the last weeks of pregnancy you may also be asked to keep track of your baby's movements. If you notice your baby's movements becoming less frequent or slowing down, or if they stop, contact your midwife or doctor immediately.

If tests show that your baby is not growing well in the womb, early delivery by induction of labour or Caesarean section (see page 101) may be recommended.

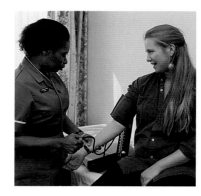

HIGH BLOOD PRESSURE AND PRE-ECLAMPSIA

During pregnancy your blood pressure will be checked at every antenatal appointment. This is because a rise in blood pressure can be the first sign of a condition known as pre-eclampsia – often called pregnancy-induced hypertension (PIH) or pre-eclamptic toxaemia (PET) – which can run in families and affects 10% of pregnancies. Your urine will also be checked for protein.

If you do have pre-eclampsia, you will probably feel perfectly well. Some women experience symptoms such as headaches, visual disturbances, swelling and abdominal pain. Pre-eclampsia can still be severe, however, without any symptoms at all. Although most cases are mild and cause no trouble, it can get worse and be serious for both mother and baby. It can cause fits in the mother (Eclampsia) and affect the baby's growth, and be life-threatening if left untreated. That is why routine antenatal checks are so important.

Pre-eclampsia usually happens towards the end of pregnancy, but problems can occur earlier. Rarely, it can happen after the birth. The earlier in pregnancy it starts, the more severe it is likely to be. If it does get worse, the treatment ranges from rest at home or in hospital, drugs to lower the high blood pressure or, occasionally early delivery of the baby.

VAGINAL BLEEDING

Bleeding from the vagina at any time in pregnancy can be a danger signal. In early pregnancy, bleeding may be a sign of an ectopic pregnancy or a miscarriage (see page 104), although many women who bleed at this time go on to have normal and successful pregnancies. If you have bleeding with pain contact your GP straight away.

Bleeding after about five months may be a sign that the placenta is implanted in the lower part of the uterus (placenta praevia) or that it has started to separate from the uterus (placental abruption). Both of these can be dangerous for you and the baby, so contact your midwife or doctor immediately.

The cells on the surface of the cervix often change in pregnancy and make it more likely to bleed, particularly after intercourse. This is called a cervical erosion. Vaginal infections can also cause a small amount of vaginal bleeding.

Some causes of vaginal bleeding are more serious than others, so it's important to find the cause straight away. The most common sort of bleeding in late pregnancy is the small amount of blood mixed with mucus, known as a 'show'. This is a sign that the cervix is changing and becoming ready for labour to start. It may happen a few days before contractions start or during labour itself. You should always report this to your doctor or midwife as soon as it occurs.

SEVERE ITCHING AND OBSTETRIC CHOLESTASIS

Although itching is very common in normal pregnancy, severe generalised itching, without a rash, particularly in the last four months of pregnancy, may be the only sign of an uncommon condition called obstetric cholestasis. This is a potentially dangerous liver disorder which seems to run in families, although it can occur without any family history. It is important to contact your doctor if you have troublesome itching because obstetric cholestasis may lead to premature labour, stillbirth or serious health problems for the baby, and to an increased risk of maternal haemorrhage after the delivery.

10 What you need for the baby

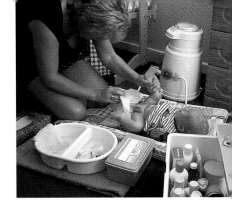

This is a list of essential items you need to get before your baby is born, and some others that you may want to think about. You may be able to borrow some of these items and then pass them on later to another baby. Look out for secondhand equipment too but do check that it is safe. Ask your health visitor if you're in doubt.

NAPPIES

CHOOSING NAPPIES

You can get terry towelling (terries) or disposable. Each has advantages and disadvantages.

Disposable nappies cost more to use but they save time and are useful if washing and drying are a problem where you live.

Terries are cheaper to use, even taking into account the cost of washing them. They are more environmentally friendly but the washing, sterilising and drying do mean more work.

Shaped, washable nappies are also available, often with a Velcro fastening.

If you do opt for terry nappies, you'll need two dozen or you'll run out. You also need:

- **nappy pins**;

- **nappy liners** – either disposable or cloth, which you can wash and use again;

- **plastic pants** – about four pairs, either tie-on or elasticated. Tie-on ones often fit small babies better;

- **a bucket with a lid and nappy sterilising powder or liquid** for sterilising nappies.

There may be a **nappy laundering** or delivery service near where you live.

CHANGING NAPPIES

You'll need:

- **cotton wool** – always choose white, and rolls are cheaper;

- **a plastic changing mat** is very useful and convenient but you can make do with a piece of waterproof sheet over an old towel;

- **baby lotion or baby wipes** – water is fine and cheap for cleaning your baby's bottom, but lotion or wipes can be convenient, especially when you're out;

- **baby barrier cream** to help prevent nappy rash – though the best way to prevent this is by changing and cleaning your baby's bottom well and often;

- **a changing bag** to carry all the nappy-changing equipment when you go out. A carrier bag will do but you can get special changing bags that include a changing mat.

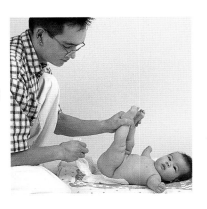

85

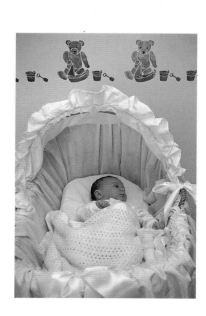

BATHING

- Any **large, clean bowl** will do as long as it's not metal. Or you can always use the sink, but remember to wrap a towel round the taps for safety.

- You need **baby soap or liquid** which can also be used on babies' hair. Ordinary toilet soap may irritate your baby's skin. It isn't necessary to use baby shampoo.

- **Two towels,** the softer the better. There's no need for special baby towels, unless you want them. Keep the towels for your baby's use only.

SAFETY

Pillows and duvets are not safe for babies less than a year old because of the risk of suffocation. Duvets can also make the baby too hot. Baby nests and quilted sleeping bags are not suitable for your baby to sleep in at any time when you are not there, again because of the danger of suffocation.

SLEEPING

For the first few months, you will need a **crib, a carry cot** or a **Moses basket**. Your baby just needs somewhere to sleep that is safe and warm and not too far away from you. You also need:

- a **firm mattress** which must fit the cot snugly, without leaving spaces round the edges – the baby could trap his or her head and suffocate. It's best if the mattress has a built-in plastic cover but, if not, you can put a waterproof sheet under the bottom sheet (never use thin plastic or a bin liner as your baby could suffocate in the loose folds);

- **sheets** to cover the mattress – you need at least four because they need to be changed so often – fitted sheets make life easy but they are quite expensive; you could use pieces of old sheet or pillow cases instead;

- several **light blankets** for safety and warmth.

COT SAFETY

Your baby will spend many hours alone in a cot so make sure it's safe.

- The mattress must fit snugly with no space for a baby's head to get stuck.

- The bars must be smooth, securely fixed and the distance between each bar should be not less than 25 mm and not more than 60 mm so that your baby's head can't become trapped.

- The cot should be sturdy.

- The moving parts should work smoothly and not allow fingers or clothing to become trapped.

- Cot bumpers are not recommended as babies can overheat or become entangled in the fastenings.

- Never leave anything with ties – bibs, clothes, etc. – in the cot in case they get caught around your baby's neck.

- If you're buying a new cot, look for the British Standard mark BS 1753.

See page 121 for more information on reducing the risk of cot death.

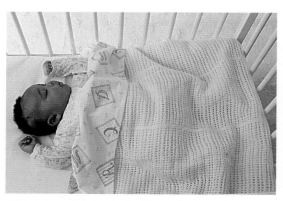

This baby is sleeping in the 'feet to foot' position (see page 121). This means that the baby's feet are right at the end of the cot to prevent the baby wriggling under the covers.

OUT AND ABOUT

Spend some time looking at what is available for getting your baby around and thinking about what will suit you best before making a choice. You could always ask other mothers what they have found useful.

- **Baby carriers** (also called slings) are attached with straps and your baby is carried in front of you. Most babies like being carried like this because they're close to you and warm. The back part of the carrier must be high enough to support your baby's head. Check that buckles and straps are secure. Older babies who can hold up their heads and whose backs are stronger (at about four months) can be carried in backpacks.

- **Pushchairs** are only suitable for young babies if they have fully reclining seats which let the baby lie flat. Wait until your baby can sit up before using any other type of pushchair. You should also consider the **weight** of the pushchair if you use public transport.

- **Prams** give your baby a lot of space to sit and lie comfortably although they take up a lot of space and cannot be used on public transport. If you have a car look for a pram which can be dismantled easily. Buy a pram harness at the same time as you will soon need it.

- **Carry cot on wheels** – your baby can sleep in the carry cot for the first few months and the cot can be attached to the frame to go out. It can also be taken in a car with appropriate restraints.

- **Three-in-one** – this is a carry cot and transporter (set of wheels) that can be converted into a pushchair when your baby outgrows the carry cot.

- **Shopping trays** which fit under the pushchair or pram can be very useful when you're out.

Before buying a pushchair or pram, etc. check that:

- *the brakes are sound;*

- *the handles are at the right height for pushing;*

- *the frame is strong enough.*

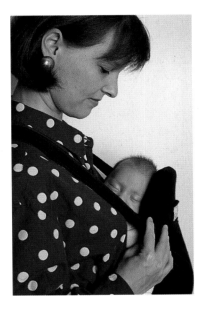

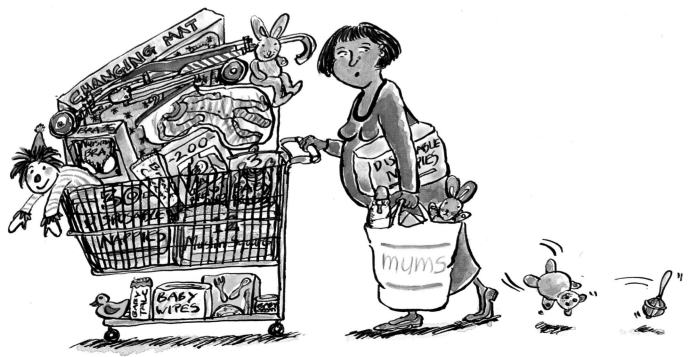

IN THE CAR

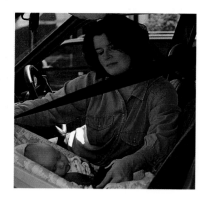

If you've got a car, you must have a safety restraint right from the start, even coming home from the hospital. It's very dangerous to carry your baby in your arms, and illegal if you are in the front seat. The best way for your baby to travel is in a rear-facing infant baby restraint (car seat) either on the front or back seat. This is held in place by the adult safety belt. Make sure it's correctly fitted. Do not place a rear-facing infant baby restraint in the front passenger seat if your car is fitted with an air bag.

Do not buy a secondhand car seat as it may have been damaged in an accident. Look for European Standard number R44/03 when you buy.

FEEDING

> ### WASHING BABY CLOTHES
>
> *If you use a washing machine, don't use enzyme (bio) powders, as they may irritate your baby's skin. Always rinse very thoroughly. Fabric softener may also cause a skin reaction.*

If you're breastfeeding you will probably want **nursing bras.** They should open at the front and have adjustable straps. Cotton is best because it allows air to circulate. If you try on bras at about 36 to 38 weeks they should fit when needed later.

A supply of **breast pads** may also be useful.

If you're going to bottle feed, you will need to get:

- **six bottles** with teats and caps;

- **sterilising equipment;**

- **a bottle brush;**

- **infant formula milk** – don't buy this too far in advance and remember to check the 'sell by date' on the pack.

CLOTHES FOR THE BABY

Babies grow very quickly. All you need for the first few weeks are enough clothes to make sure that your baby will be warm and clean. You'll probably need:

- **six stretch suits** for both day and night or four stretch suits and two nighties for the night – use socks or bootees with the nightie if it's cold;

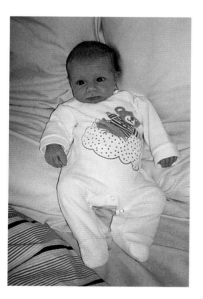

- **two cardigans,** wool or cotton rather than nylon, light rather than heavy – several light layers of clothing are best for warmth;

- **four vests;**

- **a shawl or blanket** to wrap your baby in;

- **a woolly or cotton hat, mittens, socks or bootees** for going out if the weather is cold – it's better to choose close-knitted patterns for safety;

- **a sun hat** for going out if the weather is hot or the sun is bright.

11 Labour and birth

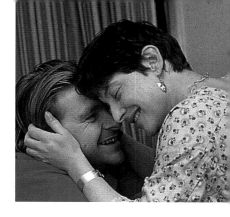

T his chapter describes a hospital birth because that is where most people have their babies, but the information will also be useful if you are having a home birth.

GETTING READY FOR THE BIRTH

PACKING FOR HOSPITAL

Pack a bag to take to hospital well in advance. Many hospitals have a printed list of what to pack. If you're having your baby at home your midwife will give you a list of things you should have ready.

You may want to include the following:

- **front-opening nighties** if you're going to breastfeed and an extra one if you're going to wear your nightie, rather than a hospital gown, during labour;

- **dressing gown** and **slippers**;

- **two or three nursing bras,** or ordinary bras if you're not breastfeeding (remember, your breasts will be much larger than usual);

- about **24 sanitary towels** (super absorbent), not tampons;

- **five or six pairs of old pants,** or disposables – you'll probably want to change often to stay fresh;

- your **washbag** with toothbrush, hairbrush, flannel, etc.;

- **towels** in a dark colour if possible;

- **change** or a **phone card** for the hospital payphone;

- a **book**, magazines, personal stereo or some knitting, for example, to help you pass the time and relax;

- a **loose comfortable outfit** to wear during the day;

- a **small bag for labour** with one or two large T-shirts, a sponge or water spray to cool you down, a personal stereo with your favourite music and anything else which you feel will make labour more pleasant for you;

- **clothes and nappies** for the baby.

For coming home

Pack loose, easy-to-wear clothes for yourself, baby clothes (including a bonnet), some nappies and a shawl or blanket to wrap the baby in.

IMPORTANT NUMBERS

Keep a list of important numbers in your handbag or near the phone. There's space for you to write them down at the beginning of this book. You need to include your hospital or midwife, your partner or birth companion, and your own hospital reference number (it will be on your card or notes) to give when you phone in. If you don't have a phone, ask neighbours for the use of theirs when the time comes.

STOCKING UP

When you come home you may not want to do much more than rest and care for your baby, so do as much planning as you can in advance. Stock up on basics such as toilet paper, sanitary pads (for you) and nappies (for the baby) and, if you have a freezer, cook some meals in advance.

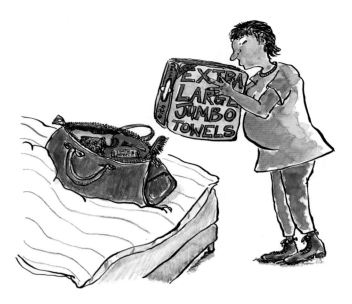

TRANSPORT

Work out how you will get to the hospital as it could be at any time of the day or night. If you're planning to go by car, make sure it's running well and that there's always enough petrol in the tank. If a neighbour has said that they will probably be able to take you, make an alternative arrangement just in case they're not in. If you haven't got a car, call an ambulance – try to do so in good time.

HOW TO RECOGNISE WHEN LABOUR STARTS

IF LABOUR STARTS EARLY

Sometimes labour starts early, even as early as 24 weeks. If this happens, get advice immediately from the hospital.

You're unlikely to mistake the signs of labour when the time really comes but, if you're in any doubt, don't hesitate to contact your hospital or midwife and ask for advice.

SIGNS THAT LABOUR IS BEGINNING

Regular contractions
You may have been feeling contractions (Braxton Hicks' contractions) – when your abdomen gets tight and then relaxes – throughout pregnancy. Lately you will have become more aware of them. When they start to come regularly, last more than 30 seconds and begin to feel stronger, labour may have started. Gradually they will become longer, stronger and more frequent.

Other signs of labour
You may or may not also have the following signs:

- **backache** or that aching, heavy feeling that some women get with their monthly period;

- a **'show'** – either before labour starts, or early in labour, the plug of mucus in the cervix, which has helped to seal the womb during pregnancy, comes away and comes out of the vagina. This small amount of sticky pink mucus is called a 'show' – you don't lose a lot of blood with a show, just a little, mixed with mucus. If you are losing more blood, it may be a sign that something is wrong, so telephone your hospital or midwife straight away;

- **the waters breaking** – the bag of water in which the baby is floating may break before labour starts (you could keep a sanitary pad (*not* a tampon) handy if you're going out, and put a plastic sheet on the bed). If the waters break before labour starts, you will notice either a slow trickle from your vagina or a sudden gush of water that you can't control – phone the hospital or your midwife, and you will probably be advised to go in at once;

- **nausea or vomiting**;

- **diarrhoea.**

PAIN RELIEF IN LABOUR

Labour is painful, so it's important to learn about all the ways you can relieve pain in labour and how your partner or labour supporter can help you. Ask your midwife or doctor to explain what is available so that you can decide what is best for you. Write down your wishes in your birth plan, but remember you may need to be flexible. You may find that you want more pain relief than you had planned and more effective pain relief may be advised to assist with delivery.

TYPES OF PAIN RELIEF

Self-help

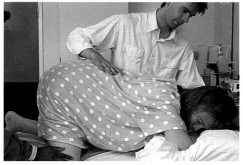

Using relaxation, breathing, keeping mobile, having a partner to support and massage you, and having confidence in your own body will all help.

'Gas and air' (Entonox)

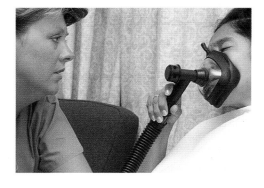

This is a mixture of oxygen and another gas called nitrous oxide. You breathe it in through a mask or mouthpiece which you hold for yourself.

You'll probably have a chance to practise using the mask or mouthpiece if you attend an antenatal class. 'Gas and air' won't remove all the pain but it can help by reducing it and making it easier to bear. Many women like it because it's easy to use and you control it yourself. The gas takes 15 to 20 seconds to work, so you breathe it in just as a contraction begins. There are no harmful side-effects for you or the baby, but it can make you feel lightheaded. Some women also find that it makes them feel sick or sleepy or unable to concentrate on what is happening. If this happens you can simply stop using it.

If you try 'gas and air' and find that it does not give you enough pain relief, you can ask for an injection as well.

TENS

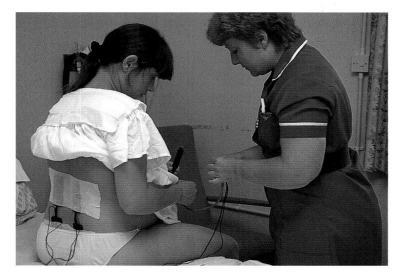

This stands for transcutaneous electrical nerve stimulation and is offered at some hospitals. In others you may need to hire a machine. It lessens the pain for many, but not all, women.

There are no known side-effects for either you or the baby and you can move around while using it.

'Gas and air seemed to work for me, provided I used it at the right time. The midwife was really good and helped me with my timing.'

'I didn't want to have any injections or anything, so my midwife told me about TENS. It sounded a bit weird when she told me what it was but, when the time came, it actually did seem to work.'

Electrodes are taped on to your back and connected by wires to a small battery-powered stimulator known as an 'obstetric pulsar'. You hold the pulsar and can give yourself small, safe amounts of current.

It is believed that TENS works by stimulating the body to increase production of its own natural painkillers, called endorphins. It also reduces the number of pain signals that are sent to the brain by the spinal cord. If you're interested in TENS you should learn how to use it in the earlier months of your pregnancy. Ask your midwife or physiotherapist.

'After the first injection, I felt wonderful, there was no pain and I was on cloud nine. But after the second one, and some gas, I felt confused and out of control, which I think extended the labour.'

Injections

Another form of pain relief is the intramuscular injection of a pain-relieving drug, usually pethidine. It takes about 20 minutes to work and the effects last between two and four hours. It will help you to relax and some women find that this lessens the pain. However, it can make some women feel very 'woozy', sick and forgetful. If it hasn't worn off when you need to push, it can make it difficult. You might prefer to ask for half a dose initially to see how it works for you. If pethidine is given too close to the time of delivery, it may affect the baby's breathing, but if it does an antidote will be given.

Epidural anaesthesia

An epidural is a special type of local anaesthetic. It numbs the nerves which carry the feelings of pain from the birth canal to the brain. So, for most women, an epidural gives complete pain relief.

'I was really scared about the pain so I chose to have an epidural. It was great — I didn't feel a thing!'

An epidural is given by an anaesthetist so, if you think you might want one, check with your midwife beforehand (perhaps when you're discussing your birth plan) about whether an anaesthetist is always available at your hospital.

While you lie on your side, anaesthetic is injected into the space between the bones in your spine through a very thin tube. It takes about 20 minutes to get the tube set up and then another 15 to 20 minutes for it to work. The anaesthetic can then be pumped in continuously or topped up when necessary.

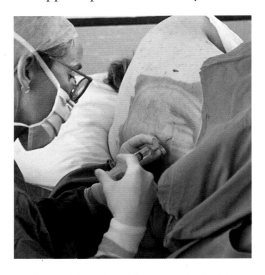

An epidural can be very helpful for those women who are having a long or particularly painful labour or who are becoming very distressed. It takes the pain of labour away for most women and you won't feel so tired afterwards. But there are disadvantages:

- your legs may feel heavy and that sometimes makes women feel rather helpless and unable to get into a comfortable position;

- you may find it difficult to pass water and a small tube called a catheter may need to be put into your bladder to help you;

- you will need to have a drip on your arm to give you fluids and help maintain adequate blood pressure;

- you won't be able to get out of bed during labour and for several hours afterwards;

- your contractions and the baby's heart will need to be monitored by a machine. This means having a belt round your abdomen and possibly a clip attached to your baby's head (see **Fetal heart monitoring**, page 96);

- if you can no longer feel your contractions, the midwife will have to tell you when to push rather than you doing it naturally – sometimes less anaesthetic is given at the end so that the effect of the epidural wears off and you can push the baby out more effectively;

- some women get backache for some time after having an epidural.

In some hospitals, a mobile or 'walking' epidural is available. The anaesthetist gives a different combination of drugs which allows you to move your legs whilst still providing effective pain relief. Ask if this is available in your hospital.

If you don't want any of these kinds of pain relief, you are free to say so. And if you decide you do want pain relief, ask for it as soon as you feel you need it, without waiting for it to be offered.

ALTERNATIVE METHODS OF PAIN RELIEF

Some mothers want to avoid the above methods of pain relief and choose acupuncture, aromatherapy, homeopathy, hypnosis, massage and reflexology. If you would like to use any of these methods, it's important to let the hospital know beforehand.

Discuss the matter with the midwife or doctor. And make sure that the practitioner you use is properly trained and experienced. For advice, contact the Institute for Complementary Medicine (see page 141).

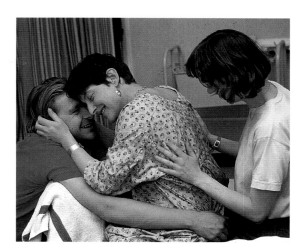

WHAT YOU CAN DO FOR YOURSELF

Fear makes pain worse and everyone feels frightened of what they don't understand or can't control. So learning about labour from antenatal classes, from your doctor or midwife, and from books like this, is an important first step.

- *Learning to relax helps you to remain calmer and birth classes can teach ways of breathing that may help with contractions.*

- *Your position can also make a difference. Some women like to kneel, walk around or rock backwards and forwards. Some like to be massaged, but others hate to be touched.*

- *Feeling in control of what is happening to you is important. You are working with the midwife and she with you, so don't hesitate to ask questions or to ask for anything you want at any time.*

- *Having a partner, friend or relative you can 'lean on', and who can support you during labour certainly helps. It has been shown to reduce the need for pain relief. But if you don't have anyone, don't worry – your midwife will give you the support you need.*

- *And finally, no one can tell you what your labour will feel like in advance. Even if you think you would prefer not to have any pain relief, keep an open mind. In some instances, it could help to make your labour more enjoyable and fulfilling.*

COPING AT THE BEGINNING

KEEPING ACTIVE

Keep active for as long as you feel comfortable. This helps the progress of the birth. Keeping active doesn't mean anything strenuous — just moving normally or walking around.

At night, try getting comfortable and relaxed and perhaps dozing off to sleep. A warm bath or shower may help you to relax. During the day, keep upright and gently active. This helps the baby to move down into the pelvis and the cervix to dilate. It's important to have something light to eat to give you energy, as labour, particularly a first one, may last 12 to 15 hours from the early stages to delivery.

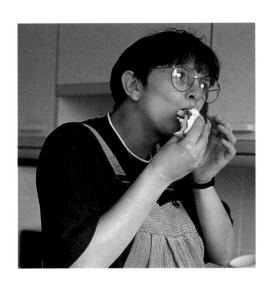

WHEN TO GO INTO HOSPITAL OR GP OR MIDWIFE UNIT

If your waters have broken you will probably be advised to go straight in. If your contractions start but your waters have not broken and you live near to the hospital or unit, wait until they are coming regularly, about five minutes apart, lasting about 60 seconds, and they feel so strong that you want to be in hospital. If the journey is likely to take a while, either because of traffic or the distance, or if this is not your first baby, go sooner and make sure you leave plenty of time to get to the hospital. Second and later babies often arrive more quickly. Don't forget to phone the hospital or unit before leaving home and remember your notes or card.

If you're at all uncertain about whether or not it is time for you to go into hospital, always telephone the hospital or unit or your midwife for advice.

HOME/DOMINO DELIVERY

Follow the procedure you have agreed with your midwife during your discussions about the onset of labour.

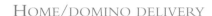

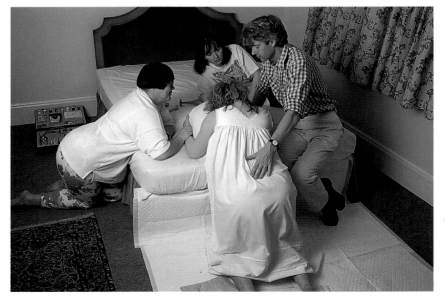

AT THE HOSPITAL

Going into hospital when you are in labour may be frightening, but attending antenatal classes and visiting the hospital during pregnancy should help. Hospitals and GP or midwife units all vary, so this is just a guide to what is likely to happen. Talk to your midwife about the way things are done at your local hospital or unit and what you would like for your birth. If your wishes can't be met, it's important to understand why (see **Birth plan**, page 37).

YOUR ARRIVAL

If you carry your own notes, take them to the hospital admissions desk. You will be taken to the labour ward, where a midwife will take you to your room and help you change into a hospital gown or a nightdress of your own. Choose an old one that is loose and preferably made of cotton because you'll feel hot during labour and won't want something tight.

EXAMINATION BY THE MIDWIFE

The midwife will ask you about what has been happening so far and will examine you. If you are having a Domino or home delivery, then this examination will take place at home. The midwife will:

- take your pulse, temperature and blood pressure and check your urine;

- feel your abdomen to check the baby's position and record or listen to your baby's heart;

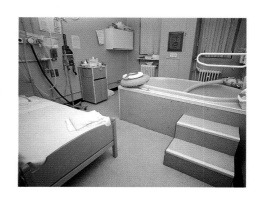

- probably do an internal examination to find out how much your cervix has opened (tell her if a contraction is coming so that she can wait until it has passed), and she will then be able to tell you how far your labour has progressed.

These checks will be repeated at intervals throughout your labour – always ask about anything you want to know. If you and your partner have made a birth plan, show your midwife so that she knows your views about your labour and can help you to achieve them. Many women find that they naturally empty their bowels before, or very early, in labour. Very occasionally, if you are constipated, a suppository may be suggested.

DELIVERY ROOMS

Some hospitals may have one or two delivery rooms decorated in a more homely way, with easy chairs and beanbags so that you can easily move around and change your position during labour. Talk to your midwife about this and write your wishes in your birth plan (see page 38).

BATH OR SHOWER

Some hospitals may offer you a bath or shower. A warm bath can be soothing in the early stages of labour. In fact, some women like to spend much of their labour in the bath as a way of easing the pain.

WATER BIRTHS

Some hospitals have birthing pools available (or you may be able to hire one) so that you can labour in water. Many women find that this helps them to relax. If labour progresses normally it may be possible to deliver the baby in the pool. This method is currently being studied, so speak to your midwife and obstetrician about the advantages and disadvantages. You'll need to make arrangements well in advance.

WHAT HAPPENS IN LABOUR

WHAT YOU CAN DO

- *You can be up and moving about if you feel like it.*

- *You may be able to have sips of water, but once in established labour you will usually be asked not to eat anything. This is mainly in case you need an anaesthetic later on. Some units, however, allow fluids and/or a light diet.*

- *If you need the midwife while she is out of the room you will be able to call her by ringing a bell.*

- *As the contractions get stronger and more painful, you can put into practice the relaxation and breathing exercises you learned during pregnancy.*

- *Your partner or friend can help by doing them with you and by rubbing your back to relieve the pain if that helps.*

There are three stages to labour. In the first stage the cervix gradually opens up (dilates). In the second stage the baby is pushed down the vagina and is born. In the third stage the placenta comes away from the wall of the womb and is also pushed out of the vagina.

THE FIRST STAGE

The dilation of the cervix

Contractions at the start of labour help to soften the cervix. Then the cervix will gradually open to about 10 cm. This is wide enough to let the baby out and is called 'fully dilated'. Sometimes the process of softening can take many hours before what midwives refer to as 'established labour'. This is when your cervix has opened (dilated) to at least 3 cm.

If you go into hospital before labour is established, you may be asked if you would prefer to go home again for a while, rather than spending many extra hours in hospital. Once labour is established, the midwife will check again from time to time to see how you are progressing. In a first labour, the time from the start of established labour to full dilation is between 6 and 12 hours. It is often quicker for later ones.

Towards the end of the first stage, you may feel that you want to push as each contraction comes. At this point, if the midwife isn't already with you, ring for her to come. The midwife will tell you to try not to push until your cervix is fully open and the baby's head can be seen. To help yourself get over the urge to push, try blowing out slowly and gently or, if the urge is too strong, in little puffs. Some people find this easier lying on their sides, or on their elbows and knees, to reduce the pressure of the baby's head on the cervix.

Fetal heart monitoring

Every baby's heart is monitored throughout labour. The midwife is watching for any marked change in the heart rate which could be a sign that the baby is distressed and that action should be taken in order to speed delivery. There are different ways of monitoring the baby's heartbeat.

- Your midwife may listen to the baby's heart intermittently with a hand-held ultrasound monitor (often called a Sonicaid). This method allows you to be free to move around in labour if you wish.

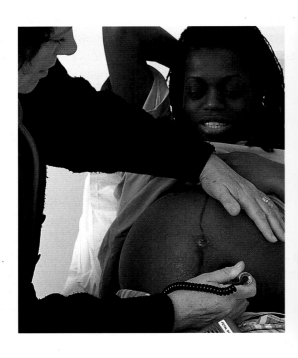

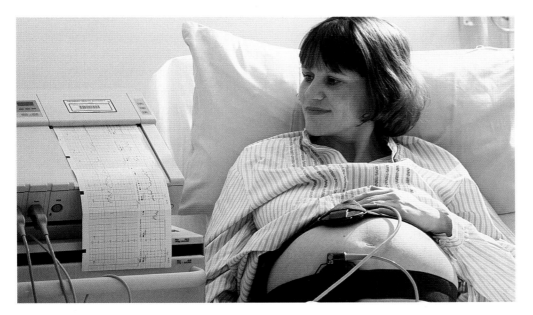

● The heartbeat and contractions may also be followed electronically through a monitor linked to a machine called a CTG. The monitor will be strapped on a belt to your tummy.

Sometimes it may be suggested that a clip is put on the baby's head so that its heart can be monitored more exactly. The clip is put on during a vaginal examination and the waters are broken if they have not already done so. Ask your midwife or doctor to explain why they feel the clip is necessary for your baby. Throughout labour the heartbeat will be followed by a bleep from the machine and a print out. You cannot easily move around. Some machines use tiny transmitters which allow you to be more mobile. Ask if this is available.

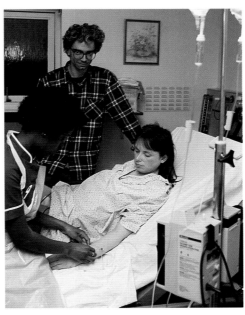

A drip may be used to speed up labour.

Speeding up labour

If your labour is slow, your doctor may recommend acceleration to get things moving. You should be given a clear explanation of why this is proposed. To start with your waters will be broken (if this has not already happened) during a vaginal examination. This is often enough to get things moving. If not, you may be offered a drip containing a hormone which will encourage contractions. If you have a drip, the hormone will be fed into a vein in your arm.

THE SECOND STAGE

The baby's birth

This stage begins when the cervix is fully dilated and lasts until the birth of the baby. Your body will tell you to push. Listen to your midwife who will guide you.

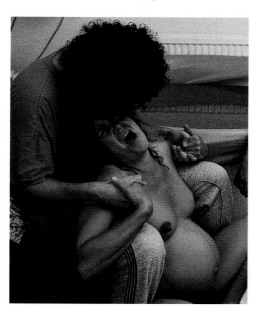

Position

Find the position that you prefer and which will make labour easier for you. You might want to remain in bed with your back propped up with pillows, or stand, sit, kneel or squat (squatting will take practice if you are not used to it). If you are very tired, you might be more comfortable lying on your side rather than your back. This is also a better position for your baby.

If you've suffered from backache in labour, kneeling on all fours might be helpful. It's up to you. Try out some of these positions at antenatal classes or at home to find out which are the most comfortable for you. Ask the midwife to help you.

Pushing

You can now start to push each time you have a contraction. Your body will probably tell you how. If not, take two deep breaths as the contractions start and push down.

Take another breath when you need to. Give several pushes until the contraction ends. As you push, try to let yourself 'open up' below. After each contraction, rest and get up strength for the next one. This stage is hard work but your midwife will help you all the time, telling you what to do and encouraging you. Your companion can also give you lots of support. Ask your midwife to tell you what is happening. This stage may take an hour or more, so it helps to know how you're doing.

The birth

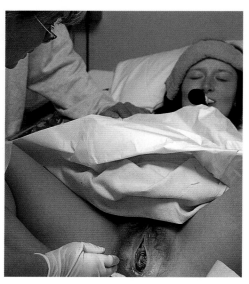

As the baby's head moves into the vaginal opening you can put your hand down to feel it, or look at it in a mirror. When about half the head can be seen, the midwife will tell you to stop pushing, to push very gently, or to puff a couple of quick short breaths blowing out through your mouth. This is so that your baby's head can be born slowly, giving the skin and muscles of the perineum (the area between your vagina and back passage) time to stretch without tearing.

Sometimes the skin of the perineum won't stretch enough and may tear. Or there may be an urgency to hurry the birth because the baby is getting short of oxygen. The midwife or doctor will then ask

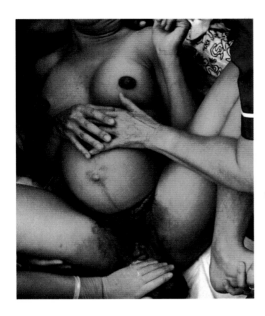

Once the baby's head is born, the body usually follows quite quickly and easily with one more push.

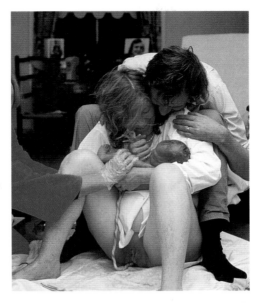

You can have your baby lifted straight on to you before the cord is cut.

Your baby may be born still covered with some of the white, greasy vernix which acts as a protection in the womb.

your permission to give you a local anaesthetic and cut the skin to make the opening bigger. This is called an episiotomy. Afterwards the cut or tear is stitched up again and heals. Once your baby's head is born, most of the hard work is over. With one more gentle push the body is born quite quickly and easily. You can ask to have the baby lifted straight on to you before the cord is cut, so that you can feel and be close to each other immediately. Then the cord is clamped and cut, the baby is dried to prevent him or her from becoming cold, and you'll be able to hold and cuddle your baby properly. Your baby may be quite messy, with some of your blood and perhaps some of the white, greasy vernix which acts as a protection in the womb still on the skin. If you prefer, you can ask the midwife to wipe your baby and wrap him or her in a blanket before your cuddle.

Sometimes some mucus has to be cleared out of a baby's nose and mouth or some oxygen given to get breathing underway. Your baby won't be kept away from you any longer than necessary.

THE THIRD STAGE

The placenta

After your baby is born, more contractions will push out the placenta. This stage can take between 20 minutes and an hour but your midwife will usually give you an injection in your thigh, just as the baby is born, which will speed it up.

The injection contains a drug called Syntometrine or Syntocinon which makes the womb contract and so helps prevent the heavy bleeding which some women may experience without it. You may prefer not to have the injection at first, but to wait and see if it is necessary. You should discuss this in advance with your midwife and make a note on your birth plan.

'All I wanted afterwards was to go to sleep.'

'I kept looking at him and thinking, "I've actually got one! He's mine! I've done it at last!"'

'It was like being drunk, I felt so special, so full of myself and what I'd done.'

A paediatrician may check your baby straight after delivery.

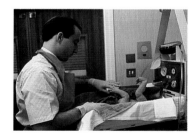

If you're breastfeeding, let your baby suckle as soon after birth as possible. Babies do suck this soon, although maybe just for a short time, or they may just like to feel the nipple in the mouth. It helps with breastfeeding later on and it also helps your womb to contract.

AFTERWARDS

If you've had a deep tear or an episiotomy, it will be sewn up. If you have had an epidural you will not feel this. Otherwise you should be offered a local anaesthetic injection. If it is sore during this repair, then say so; it is the only way that the midwife or doctor will know that they are hurting you. Small tears and grazes are often left to heal without stitches because they frequently heal better this way.

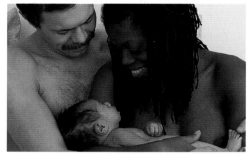

Your baby will be examined, weighed and possibly measured and given a band with your name on it. The midwife will then help you to wash and freshen up. Then you should have some time alone with your baby and your partner, just to be together quietly and meet your new baby properly. If you find this doesn't happen and you would like some time alone, ask for it.

SPECIAL CASES

LABOUR THAT STARTS TOO EARLY (PREMATURE LABOUR)

About one baby in every ten will be born before the 37th week of pregnancy. In most cases labour starts by itself, either with contractions or with the sudden breaking of the waters or a show (see page 90). About one early baby in three is induced (see page 101) or delivered by Caesarean section (see pages 101–2) because doctors feel that early delivery is necessary for your own or the baby's safety.

If your baby is likely to be delivered early, you will be admitted to a hospital with specialist facilities for premature babies. Not all hospitals have facilities for the care of very premature babies, so it may be necessary to transfer you and your baby to another unit, either before delivery or immediately afterwards. If contractions start well before you are due, the doctors may be able to use drugs to stop your contractions temporarily. You will probably be advised to have injections of steroids that will help to mature your baby's lungs so that he or she is better able to breathe after the birth. This

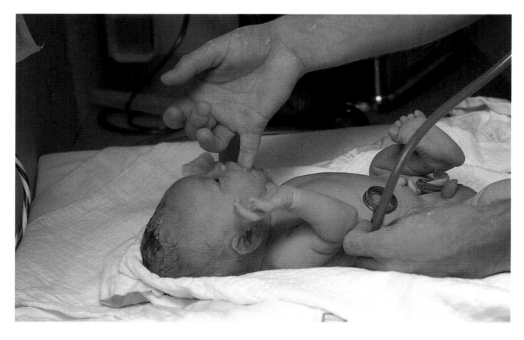

treatment takes about 24 hours to work.

If you have any reason to think that your labour may be starting early, get in touch with your hospital or midwife at once so that arrangements can be made.

BABIES BORN LATE

Pregnancy normally lasts about 40 weeks, that is 280 days from the first day of your last period. Most women will go into labour within a week either side of this date. If your labour does not start, the doctor will want to keep a careful check on your baby's health. This is often referred to as 'monitoring'. If there is any evidence that your baby is not doing well, or if you are overdue by a week or two, the doctor will suggest that labour is induced (see below).

INDUCTION

Sometimes labour must be started artificially. This is called induction. Labour may be induced if there is any sort of risk to the mother's or baby's health – for example, if the mother has high blood pressure or if the baby is failing to grow and thrive. Induction is always planned in advance, so you will be able to talk over the advantages and disadvantages with your doctor and midwife and find out why it is thought suitable in your particular case.

Contractions can be started by inserting a pessary or gel into the vagina, or by a hormone drip in the arm. Sometimes both are used. Induction of labour may take a while, particularly if the neck of the womb (cervix) needs to be softened with pessaries or gels. Once labour starts it should proceed normally.

FORCEPS DELIVERY OR VACUUM EXTRACTION

If the baby needs to be helped out of the vagina – perhaps because the contractions aren't strong enough, because the baby has got into an awkward position or is becoming distressed, or because you have become too exhausted – then forceps or vacuum extraction (sometimes called Ventouse) will be used.

A local anaesthetic will usually be given to numb the birth canal, if you haven't already had an epidural or spinal anaesthetic.

Forceps are placed round the baby's head by an obstetrician and with gentle firm pulling the baby can be born. With vacuum delivery, a shallow rubber or metal cap is fitted to the baby's head by suction. You can help by pushing when the obstetrician asks you to. Sometimes you will find red marks on your baby's head where the forceps have been or a swelling from the vacuum. They will soon fade.

An episiotomy (see page 98) is nearly always needed for a forceps delivery.

Your partner or companion should be able to stay with you if you wish.

CAESAREAN SECTION

There are situations where the safest option for either you or your baby, or both, is to have a Caesarean section. As a Caesarean section involves major surgery, it will only be performed where there is a real clinical need for this type of delivery. The baby is delivered by cutting through the abdomen and then into the womb. The cut is usually done crossways and low down, just below the bikini line. It is usually hidden when your pubic hair grows back again.

HEPATITIS B

Some people carry the virus in their blood without actually having the disease itself. If a pregnant mother has hepatitis B, or catches it during pregnancy, she can pass it on to her child. The child may not be ill but has a high chance of becoming a carrier and developing liver disease later in life. Babies born to infected mothers should receive a course of vaccine to prevent them from getting hepatitis B and becoming a carrier. The first dose is given within 24 hours of birth, and two more doses are given at one and two months with a booster dose at twelve months old.

'I wasn't elated or anything like that. I think it had all been too much like hard work to feel much after.'

'I was relieved. I was delighted about the baby, but I was more relieved than anything – that it was over, and we'd come through, and everything was fine'.

(A FATHER)

101

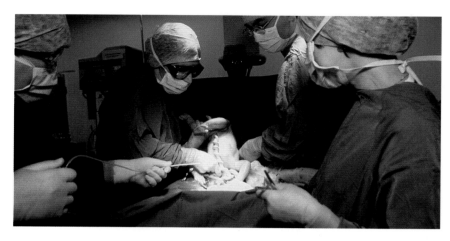

A Caesarean under an epidural anaesthetic.

NEXT TIME

Once a Caesarean always a Caesarean?

If you have your first baby by Caesarean section, this does not necessarily mean that any future baby will be delivered in this way. Vaginal birth after a previous Caesarean can and does happen. This will depend on your own particular circumstances (see page 129). You can discuss your hopes and plans for any other deliveries with your doctor or midwife.

A Caesarean section may be 'elective' (that is, planned in advance) or 'emergency'. An elective Caesarean may be recommended if labour is judged to be dangerous for you or the baby. An emergency Caesarean may be necessary if complications develop and delivery needs to be quick. This may be before or during labour. Sometimes the cervix does not dilate fully during labour and an emergency Caesarean will be suggested but, providing you and the baby are well, there is no need to proceed with great haste.

Whenever a Caesarean is suggested, your doctor should explain why it is necessary and any possible side-effects. Do not hesitate to ask questions.

Where possible, the operation is performed under epidural anaesthesia (see page 92) or the similar spinal anaesthetic. A general anaesthetic is sometimes used, particularly when the baby needs to be delivered very quickly or if there are technical problems, but this increases the risks for you and the baby. This is why epidural and spinal anaesthetics are recommended.

If you have an epidural, you will be awake throughout the operation but you won't feel pain, just some tugging and pulling and wetness when the waters break. A screen will be put across your chest so that you cannot see what is being done. The doctors will talk to you and let you know what is happening.

The operation takes about 30 to 40 minutes. One advantage of an epidural or spinal anaesthetic is that you are awake at the moment of delivery and you can see and hold your baby immediately. Most hospitals are willing to let your partner be present at a Caesarean under epidural or spinal so that they can give you lots of support and welcome the baby at birth. Please ask.

After a Caesarean you will be uncomfortable for a few days, as you would expect to be after any major surgery. It will be difficult to sit up or stand up straight and it will hurt to laugh. You will have to stay in hospital a bit longer, about five to seven days, but this will depend on your condition. You will also have to take it easy once you are home and you will need help. You shouldn't lift anything heavy or drive a car for six weeks. Your doctor or midwife will advise you on how much you can do. Postnatal exercises are especially important after a Caesarean to get your muscles working again, but take things at a gentle pace. The midwife or hospital physiotherapist will tell you when you should begin them. You can also contact the Caesarean Support Network for information and support (see page 141).

BREECH BIRTH

A breech birth is when a baby is born bottom first. Your obstetrician and midwife will discuss with you the best and safest way for your breech baby to be born. They may arrange an ultrasound scan to assess how big your baby is. They may advise a Caesarean section, or they may encourage vaginal delivery depending upon your individual circumstances. Ultimately, the decision is yours.

A vaginal breech delivery is a little more complicated, than the usual 'head first' delivery. An epidural is usually recommended and forceps are often used to deliver the baby's head (see page 101). In some units you will be offered the option of an external cephalic version (ECV). The baby is turned into the usual head down position (cephalic) by pressing on the woman's tummy.

TWINS

If you are expecting twins, labour may start early because the womb becomes very stretched with two babies. More people will usually be present at the birth – for example, a midwife, an obstetrician, and usually two paediatricians, one for each baby.

The process of labour is the same but the babies will be closely monitored, usually by using an electronic monitor (see page 96). You will be given a drip in case it is needed later and an epidural will often be recommended. Once the first baby has been born, the midwife or doctor will check the position of the second by feeling your abdomen and doing a vaginal examination. If the second baby is in a good position to be born, the waters surrounding the baby will be broken and the second baby should be born very soon after the first because the cervix is already fully dilated. If contractions stop after the first birth, hormones will be added to the drip to restart them.

If you're expecting twins or more babies, you might like to contact the Twins and Multiple Births Association (TAMBA) for advice and support (see page 142).

WHAT YOUR COMPANION CAN DO

Whoever your labour partner is – the baby's father, a close friend, or a relative – there are quite a few practical things that he or she can do to help you, although probably none of them are as important as just being with you. You can't know in advance what your labour is going to be like or how each of you will cope. But there are many ways in which a partner can help.

Your labour partner can:

- keep you company and help pass the time in the early stages;

- hold your hand, wipe your face, give you sips of water, massage your back and shoulders, help you move about or change position, or anything else that helps and comforts you as your labour progresses and your contractions get stronger;

- remind you how to use relaxation and breathing techniques, perhaps breathing with you if it helps;

- support your decisions about, for example, pain relief;

- help you make it clear to the midwife or doctor what help you need – and the other way round – which can help you to feel much more in control of the situation;

- as your baby is born, tell you what is happening, because you can't see what is going on for yourself.

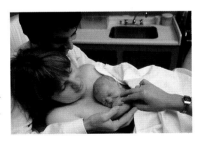

For very many couples, being together during labour and welcoming their baby together is an experience that they can't begin to put into words. And many fathers who have seen their baby born and who have played a part themselves say they feel much closer to the child from the very start.

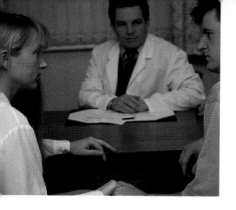

12 When pregnancy goes wrong

Unfortunately, not all pregnancies end well. For a few, pregnancy ends with a miscarriage or with the death of the baby. This chapter describes some of the things that can go wrong. If your pregnancy ends in this way, then you will need both information and support. Talk to the people close to you about how you feel and to your doctor, midwife or health visitor about what has happened and why. Sometimes it is easier to talk to someone outside your immediate circle. Organisations offering information and support are listed on page 141.

ECTOPIC PREGNANCY

After fertilisation the egg should move down into the womb to develop. Sometimes it gets stuck in the fallopian tube and begins to grow there. This is called an 'ectopic' or 'tubal' pregnancy. The fertilised egg can't develop properly and has to be removed in an operation.

A common cause of an ectopic pregnancy is some sort of blockage in the fallopian tube, possibly as a result of an infection. Warning signs start soon after a missed period. They are a severe pain on one side, low down in the abdomen, vaginal bleeding or brown discharge, and sometimes feeling faint, and women should see their doctor immediately.

Talk to your doctor to find out why it happened and whether your chances of conceiving a baby have been affected. One organisation which can offer support is called Child (see page 141).

MISCARRIAGE

If a pregnancy ends in the first six months it is known as a miscarriage. Miscarriages are quite common in the first three months of pregnancy. Probably at least one in six clinically recognised pregnancies ends this way. At this stage a miscarriage usually happens because there is something wrong with the baby. A later miscarriage may be due to the placenta not developing or working properly, or the cervix being weak and opening too early in the pregnancy.

An early miscarriage can be rather like a period, with bleeding and a similar sort of aching pain, maybe occurring on and off, happening at the time when a period would have been due. With a later miscarriage, bleeding is likely to be accompanied by pains that feel more like the pains that come with labour.

If you bleed or begin to have pains, you should contact the person who is giving you antenatal care, either at the hospital or your GP's surgery. You may be told to lie down quietly or to come into hospital immediately. Sometimes the bleeding stops by itself and your pregnancy will carry on quite normally. But if a miscarriage is going to happen, there is very little that anyone can do to stop it.

After a miscarriage, you may have a 'D and C' (that is, dilatation and curettage) to empty the womb. This is done under anaesthetic. The cervix is gently widened and the lining of the womb scraped or sucked away. The cervix narrows again afterwards.

AFTERWARDS

One miscarriage will not affect your chances of having a baby in the future. Even after three miscarriages you still stand a good chance of carrying a baby to term. If you have three or more miscarriages, you should be referred for further investigations. In some cases, all investigations will be normal and no precise cause found.

A miscarriage can be very difficult to come to terms with. You may feel disappointed, angry, or even guilty, wondering what you did wrong. Some people fear that the miscarriage may have been caused by making love, though this is extremely unlikely. In fact, whatever the cause, it is very rarely anyone's fault.

You will almost certainly feel a sense of loss. You need time to grieve over the lost baby just as you would over the death of anyone close to you, especially if the miscarriage has happened later in pregnancy. Many people find it helps to have something to remember their baby by. In early pregnancy you might be able to have a picture of a scan. After about four months you could ask for a photograph of the baby. If your miscarriage is very late you may be able to see and hold your baby, if you wish, as well as having a photograph. Talking also helps. Talk about your feelings with your partner and those close to you. The Miscarriage Association (see page 142) can give you information and put you in touch with other women who have experienced a miscarriage.

TERMINATION

If tests show that your baby has a serious abnormality you may consider whether or not to end your pregnancy (see page 57). It is important to find out as much information as you can from the doctor about the particular condition and how it may affect your baby, so that you can make a decision that is right for you and your family.

You will probably be very shocked when you are first told the diagnosis by the consultant and may not be able to take very much in. You may need to go back and talk again, preferably accompanied by your partner or someone close to you. You will also need to spend time talking things through with your partner or with others close to you.

An early termination, before 12 to 14 weeks, will usually be done under a general anaesthetic. For a later termination you will probably go through labour as this is usually the safest way for you. You may wish to think beforehand about whether you want to see and perhaps even hold your baby and give your baby a name. It can make the baby more real for you and your family and help you to grieve. If you don't wish to see your baby, it's still a good idea to ask hospital staff to take a

*A funeral or some other way
of saying goodbye may be a
very important part of
coming to terms with your
loss, however early it
happens. If your baby
dies after 24 weeks of
pregnancy the hospital must
provide a death certificate
and arrange a burial or
cremation. If you would like
to arrange it yourself or
organise a service you can do
that. Just speak to the ward
staff and they will tell
you what the arrangements
are in your hospital.*

photograph for you. You may find this comforting at a later date.

You may find your feelings quite hard to cope with after a termination, whether it has been in early or late pregnancy. It will help to talk about them. If you would like to talk to people who have undergone a similar experience you can contact ARC (Antenatal Results and Choices) (see page 142).

LOSING A BABY

In the UK about 4000 babies every year are stillborn – the baby is already dead when it is born. About the same number die soon after birth. Often the causes of these deaths are not known.

If you lose a baby like this, you are likely to feel very shocked. But you and your partner may find it comforting to see and hold your baby and give your baby a name. You may also like to have a photograph of your baby and to keep some mementos such as a lock of hair or the shawl the baby was wrapped in. All this can help you and your family to remember your baby as a real person and can, in time, help in coming to terms with your loss. Many hospitals have a bereavement counsellor who will

help you to find the best way for you and your partner to cope with your loss.

One of the first questions you are likely to ask is why your baby died. The doctors and midwives may not know. A post-mortem examination is usually advised and this may help to find out, although it doesn't always provide the answer. Most hospitals will offer you an appointment with the consultant who can explain to you what is known. If you are not offered an appointment, you can ask for one.

It may also help to talk about your feelings with other parents who have lost a baby in a similar way. SANDS (the Stillbirth and Neonatal Death Society) is an organisation that can put you in touch with other parents who can offer friendly help (see page 142).

You may well want to arrange a cremation, funeral or service. You should be able to do so. If the baby was lost after 24 weeks, the loss will need to be officially registered as either a death or a stillbirth. If you want to arrange a funeral or cremation and your baby was lost before 24 weeks, you will need a certificate from the hospital. Talk to your midwife or doctor about what you want to do and to find out what arrangements are available locally. You could also consult the hospital chaplain or rabbi or your own religious adviser.

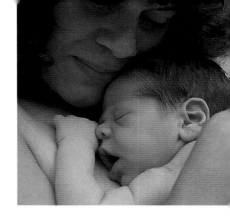

13 The first days with your new baby

In the first few days after the birth, you and your baby are beginning to get to know each other. Don't feel you have to make a great effort. Just have your baby close to you as much as you can.

Partners also need plenty of opportunity to handle the baby and feel close. Many fathers feel a little left out, especially if they have to leave you and the baby in hospital and return to an empty home. They may need support and encouragement to get involved, but the more you can both hold and cuddle your baby the more confident you'll all feel.

YOU

You may feel tired for the first few days, so make sure you get plenty of rest. Even just walking and moving about can seem like hard work. If you've had stitches they'll feel sore and you may feel worried about going to the toilet.

Once your breasts start to fill with milk they may feel uncomfortable or painful for a day or so. If you're breastfeeding, it will help to feed your baby as often as he or she needs (see page 69). You might also like to apply a warm cloth just before a feed to help relieve the engorgement. If you intend to bottle feed from the start you needn't do anything but, on the third or fourth day, your breasts may be tender as the milk is still being produced. Wearing a firm, supportive bra may help. Speak to your midwife if you are very uncomfortable.

For a lot of mothers the excitement and the pleasure of the new baby far outweigh any problems. But some do begin to feel low (see page 117) or rather depressed, especially if they are very tired or feel that they are not making any progress or can't look after their baby as they would like.

Giving birth is an emotional and tiring experience and your hormones change dramatically in the first few days. Some women feel rather weepy around the third day, especially if the labour was difficult, or if they are very tired or have other worries. This is known as the 'baby blues'. Some women worry because they don't love their baby immediately but, as with any relationship, it's not always love at first sight. You may just need to give yourself time – you can still care for your baby and provide all the warmth and security he or she needs.

'I don't think I'll ever forget those first few days. Feeling so happy. Though I don't know why. I couldn't sleep, the ward was so noisy. I was sore. I couldn't move about very well. I missed Alan and home. But I felt happier than I can ever begin to say.'

'I couldn't believe it. I'd never been much of a one for babies. And Dean wasn't even a pretty baby, not at first. Very spotty and blotchy. But he was perfect to me. He bowled me over.'

'I felt awful. I was so tired, on top of everything else. But there was one thing about it. Bob got to know the baby much better than he would have done if I'd been more on top. He was holding her and cuddling her right from the start.'

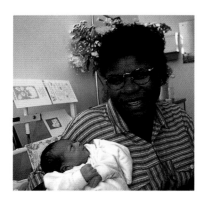

BEING IN HOSPITAL

If you have your baby in hospital, you'll probably be moved to the postnatal ward after the birth to be with other mothers who have also had their babies. Some mothers enjoy their stay in hospital and find it restful and easy. Others find it tiring and rather stressful. It depends on how you're feeling, whether you like the company of other mothers or miss your privacy, and on how the ward is organised. In any case, your stay in hospital, if your delivery is uncomplicated, is likely to be short.

It helps if you've discussed your postnatal care with your midwife during pregnancy so you know what to expect. Any preferences can then be recorded on your birth plan (see page 38) so that staff on the postnatal ward will be aware of your wishes.

You're likely to need quite a lot of help and advice with your first baby. The midwives are there to guide and support you as well as checking that you are recovering from the birth. Don't hesitate to ask for help if you need it. If you do have a problem with the way things are organised in hospital, talk it over with one of the staff. Perhaps a change can be made.

If all is going well with both you and the baby, then most hospitals will probably give you the option of going home after 48 hours or even earlier, even if it's your first baby.

The community midwife will visit you at home and continue to help you to care for yourself and your baby. You will need to make sure that your partner or someone else can be there to help you at home and do the cooking and housework.

STITCHES

If you've had stitches, bathing the area often will help healing. Use a bath, shower or cotton wool and plain warm water. After bathing,

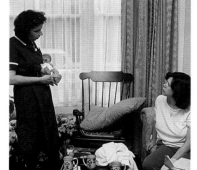

dry the vulva carefully. Pelvic floor exercises can also help healing (see page 16). If the stitches are sore and uncomfortable, tell your midwife as she may be able to recommend treatment. Painkilling tablets will also help. If there is swelling and bruising, it may be possible to have some ultrasound treatment from the physiotherapist. In any case, remember to sit down gently and lie on your side rather than your back to start with.

The thought of passing urine can be a bit frightening at first because of the soreness and because you can't seem to feel what you are doing. Sometimes it's easier to pass urine while sitting in a bowl of water or a warm bath. The water dilutes the urine so that it doesn't sting. If you really find it impossible to pass urine, tell your midwife. Also drink lots of water to dilute the urine.

You probably won't need to open your bowels for a few days after the birth but it's important not to let yourself become constipated. Eat fresh fruit, vegetables, salad and brown bread, and drink plenty of water. This should mean that when you do open your bowels you will pass a stool more easily. Whatever it may feel like, it's very unlikely that you will break the stitches or open up the cut or tear again, but it might feel better if you hold a pad of clean tissue over the stitches when you are trying to pass a stool. Avoid straining for the first few days. Sometimes stitches have to be taken out but usually they just dissolve after a week or so, by which time the cut or tear will have healed.

PILES

Piles (see page 81) are very common after delivery but they usually disappear within a few days. Eat plenty of fresh fruit, vegetables, salad, brown bread and wholegrain cereals, and drink plenty of water. This should make it easier and less painful when you pass a stool. Try not to push or strain as this will make the piles worse. Let the midwife know if you feel very uncomfortable. She will be able to give you an ointment to soothe them.

BLEEDING

After the birth you will lose blood and discharge from the vagina. The loss will probably be quite heavy at first which is why you will need super absorbent sanitary towels. Do **not** use tampons until after your postnatal check since they can cause infections in the early weeks after the birth. During breastfeeds you may notice that the discharge is more red or heavier. You may also have 'after pains'. These are both because feeding causes the womb to contract. They are a good sign that everything inside you is going back to normal. Bleeding often becomes heavier around seven to ten days after delivery but, if you find you are losing blood in large clots, you should save these towels to show the midwife as you may need some treatment. Gradually, the discharge will become a brownish colour and may continue for some weeks, getting less and less.

If you're breastfeeding you may not have another period until you stop feeding or even for some weeks or months after that. If you are not breastfeeding, your first period might start as early as a month after the birth. But it could be much later. You can become pregnant before your period starts even if you are breastfeeding, so make sure you decide on a reliable form of contraception before you and your partner make love again (see page 117).

YOUR SHAPE

Your breasts will be larger at first and while you are breastfeeding regularly. You need to wear a supportive nursing bra if you are breastfeeding. If you are not breastfeeding your breasts will reduce in size in a week or so.

Your abdomen will seem quite baggy after delivery. Despite having delivered your baby plus the placenta and a lot of fluid, you will still be quite a lot bigger than you were before pregnancy. This is partly because your muscles have stretched. If you eat a balanced diet and exercise, your shape should soon return to normal. Breastfeeding helps because it makes the womb contract. Sometimes, because this is happening, you may feel a quite painful twinge in your abdomen or period-type pain while you are feeding. Breastfeeding also uses up more calories so it can help you to lose some of the weight gained in pregnancy. Some women do not return to their normal weight until after they have finished breastfeeding.

Postnatal exercises (see page 115) will help to tone up the muscles of your pelvic floor and tummy and help you find your waist again! They will also get you moving and feeling generally fitter. You may be able to attend a postnatal exercise class while you are in hospital and afterwards. Ask your midwife or physiotherapist.

It is quite common after having a baby to find it difficult to control your bladder if you laugh, or move suddenly, and to leak some water. Pelvic floor exercises (see page 16) will help with this. If the problem persists after three months, see your doctor who may refer you to a physiotherapist.

'That first week was nothing but problems. One thing after another, first me and then the baby. Everybody was very helpful, but it was still a week or two before I got sorted out.'

CONTRACEPTION

(See also page 117)
Before you leave hospital, a midwife or doctor will probably talk to you about contraception. If this doesn't happen, you may want to ask. Although it may seem very early to be thinking about making love again, it can be easier to sort out any questions about contraception while you are in hospital rather than later on.

RUBELLA

If you were not immune to rubella (German measles) when tested early in your pregnancy, you will probably be offered immunisation before you leave hospital or shortly afterwards by your GP. If this doesn't happen, ask. This is a good opportunity to get it done. You should not get pregnant again for one month after the injection.

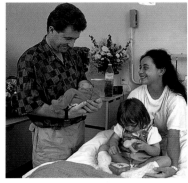

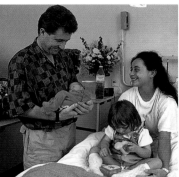

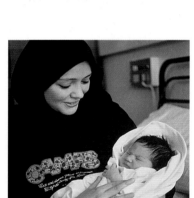

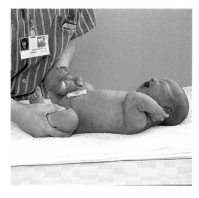

RHESUS NEGATIVE MOTHERS

If your blood group is rhesus negative and your partner's is rhesus positive, blood samples will be taken after delivery to see whether your baby is rhesus positive and whether you need an injection to protect your next baby from anaemia. If so, the injection should be given within 72 hours of delivery. Check with one of the doctors or midwives what should happen in your particular case.

YOUR BABY

Soon after birth you'll be able to look properly at your baby and notice every detail – the colour and texture of the hair, the shape of the hands and feet, and the different expressions on your baby's face. If you notice anything that worries you, however small, ask your doctor or midwife. Your baby will be examined by a doctor to make sure everything is all right. It's a good time to ask any questions you might have.

THE NAVEL

Shortly after birth the midwife will clamp the umbilical cord close to your baby's navel with a plastic clip. She then cuts the cord, leaving a small bit of cord with the clamp attached. The cord will take about a week to dry out and drop off. Keep the navel clean and dry until this happens. The midwife will show you how. If you notice any bleeding from the navel, tell your midwife, health visitor or doctor.

GUTHRIE TEST

About a week after birth, your midwife will ask to take a tiny sample of blood from your baby's heel. This is to test for rare but potentially serious illnesses. All babies are tested for phenylketonuria (a metabolic disorder) and hypothyroidism (low thyroid hormone). In some areas babies are tested for blood abnormalities like sickle cell disease and thalassaemia (see page 54). All these tests are done from a single blood sample.

VITAMIN K

We all need vitamin K to make our blood clot properly so that we won't bleed too easily. Some newborn babies have too little vitamin K. Although this is rare, it can cause them to bleed dangerously into the brain. To prevent this, you should be offered vitamin K which will be given to your baby. We don't yet know which is the safest way of giving vitamin K, whether by injection or by mouth. Your doctor or midwife will help you to choose the method you prefer.

THE FONTANELLE

On the top of your baby's head near the front, is a diamond-shaped patch where the skull bones haven't yet fused together. This is called the fontanelle. It will probably be a year or more before the bones close over it. You may notice it moving as your baby breathes. You needn't worry about touching it. There is a tough layer of membrane under the skin.

BUMPS AND BRUISES

It's quite common for a newborn baby to have some swelling and bruises on the head, and perhaps to have bloodshot eyes. This is just the result of the squeezing and pushing that is part of being born and will soon disappear. But if you are at all worried, you can always ask your midwife.

BIRTHMARKS AND SPOTS

Once you begin to look closely at your baby, you'll probably find a variety of little marks and spots, mainly on the head and face, or sometimes larger marks. Most of them will go away eventually. Ask the doctor who examines your baby if they will disappear completely. Most common are the little pink or red marks some people call 'stork bites'. These V-shaped marks on the forehead and upper eyelids gradually fade, though it may be some months before they disappear. Marks on the nape of the neck can go on much longer, but they will be covered by hair.

Strawberry marks are quite common. They are dark red and slightly raised. They sometimes appear a few days after birth and gradually get bigger. They may take a while to go away, but usually they will go away eventually.

Spots and rashes are very common in newborn babies and may come and go. But if you also notice a change in your baby's behaviour, for example if your baby is not feeding properly or is very sleepy or very irritable, you should tell your doctor or midwife immediately.

BREASTS AND GENITALS

Quite often a newborn baby's breasts are a little swollen and ooze some milk, whether the baby is a boy or a girl. Girls also sometimes bleed a bit or have a white, cloudy discharge from the vagina. All this is as a result of hormones passing from the mother to the baby before birth and is no cause for concern. The genitals of male and female newborn babies often appear rather swollen but will look in proportion with their bodies in a few weeks.

JAUNDICE

On about the third day after birth, some babies develop a yellow colour to their skin and a yellowness in the whites of their eyes because of mild jaundice. This usually fades within ten days or so. But a baby who becomes badly jaundiced may need treatment (see page 113).

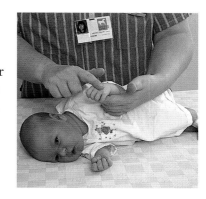

WHAT A NEWBORN BABY CAN DO

There is one important skill that babies don't have to learn. They are born knowing how to suck. During the first few days they learn to coordinate their sucking and their breathing.

Newborn babies also automatically turn towards a nipple or teat if it is brushed against one cheek and they will open their mouths if their upper lip is stroked. They can also grasp things (like your finger) with either hands or feet and they will make stepping movements if they are held upright on a flat surface. All these automatic responses except sucking, are lost within a few months, and your baby will begin to make controlled movements instead.

Newborn babies can use all their senses. They will look at people and things, especially if they are near, and particularly at people's faces. They will enjoy gentle touch, and the sound of a soothing voice and they will react to bright light and noise. Very soon they will also know their mother's special smell.

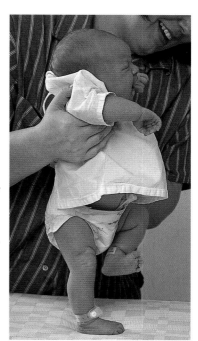

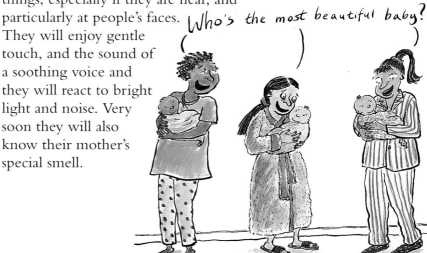

Who's the most beautiful baby?

111

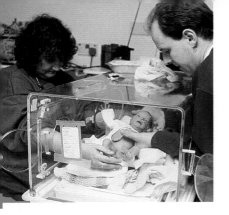

14 Babies who need special care

Some babies need special care in hospital, sometimes on the ordinary postnatal ward and sometimes in a Neonatal Unit (NNU), also known as a Special Care Baby Unit (SCBU) or Neonatal Intensive Care Unit (NICU). Babies who may need special care include:

- babies who are born early – babies born earlier than 34 weeks may need extra help breathing, feeding and keeping warm, and the earlier they are born the more help they are likely to need;

- babies who are very small or who have life-threatening conditions, usually affecting their breathing, heart and circulation;

- babies born to diabetic mothers, or babies where the delivery has been very difficult, may need to be kept under close observation for a time;

- babies with very marked jaundice;

- babies awaiting or recovering from complex surgery.

CONTACT WITH YOUR BABY

All babies need cuddling and touching, whether they are in the ward close by you or in an NNU. If your baby is in an NNU, you and your partner should try to be with your baby as much as possible. Encourage other members of your family to visit too, to get to know the baby, if this is possible. When you first go into the NNU you may be put off by all the machines and apparatus. Ask the nurse to explain what everything is for and to show you how to handle your baby.

FEEDING

Feeding is especially important for premature babies. Those who get some of their mother's milk do better, so think seriously about breastfeeding. Even if you can't stay with your baby all the time, you can express milk for the nurses to give while you are away. Some small babies can't suck properly at first and are fed by a fine tube which is passed through the nose or mouth into the stomach. You and your partner can still touch and probably hold your baby. The tube isn't painful, so you needn't worry about it being in the way or hurting your baby.

INCUBATORS

Babies who are very tiny are nursed in incubators rather than cots to keep them warm. But you can still have a lot of contact with your baby. Some incubators have open tops but, if not, you can put your hands through the holes in the side of the incubator to stroke and touch your baby. You can talk to your baby too. This is important for both of you. You may be asked to wear a gown and mask. Carefully wash and thoroughly dry your hands before touching your baby.

NEWBORN BABIES WITH JAUNDICE

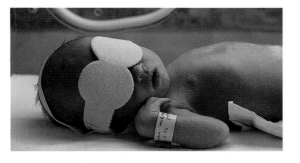

Jaundice in newborn babies is common because their livers are immature. Severely jaundiced babies may be treated by phototherapy. The baby is undressed and put under a very bright light, usually with a soft mask over the eyes. It may be possible for your baby to have phototherapy by your bed so that you don't have to be separated. This treatment may continue for several days, with breaks for feeds, before the jaundice clears up. In some cases, if the jaundice gets worse, an exchange transfusion of blood may be needed. Some babies have jaundice because of liver disease and need different treatment. A blood test before phototherapy is started checks for liver disease.

BABIES WITH JAUNDICE AFTER TWO WEEKS

Many babies are jaundiced for up to two weeks following birth. This is common in breastfed babies and usually it's normal and does no harm. It is not a reason to stop breastfeeding. But it's important to ensure that all is well if your baby is still jaundiced **after** two weeks. You should see your doctor within a day or two. This is particularly important if your baby's stools are pale. A simple urine test will distinguish between 'breast milk' jaundice, which will resolve itself, or jaundice which may need urgent treatment.

A BABY WITH DISABILITIES

If your baby is disabled in some way, you will be coping with a muddle of different feelings – love mixed with fear, pity mixed with anger. You will also need to cope with the feelings of others – your partner, relations and friends – as they come to terms with the fact that your baby is different. More than anything else at this time you will need to have a person or people to whom you can talk about how you feel and information about your baby's immediate and future prospects.

There are a number of people to whom you can turn for help – your own GP, a paediatrician at your hospital, or your health visitor. Once you are at home you can contact your social services department for information about local voluntary or statutory organisations. On page 141 you will find a list of organisations which can offer help and advice. Many are self-help groups run by parents. Talking to other parents with similar experiences can often be the most effective help.

On page 141 you will find a list of organisations which can offer help and advice.

WORRIES AND EXPLANATIONS

Always ask about the treatment your baby is being given and why, if it's not explained to you. It is important that you understand what is happening so that you can work together with hospital staff to ensure that your baby receives the best possible care. It is natural to feel anxious if your baby is having special care. Talk over any fears or worries with the staff caring for your baby.

The consultant paediatrician will probably arrange to see you, but you can also ask for an appointment if you wish. The hospital social worker may be able to help with practical problems.

113

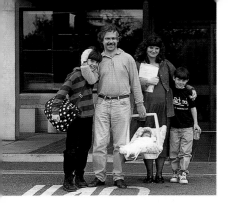

15 The early weeks: you

Going home from hospital can be very exciting, but you may feel nervous too without the hospital staff on call to help you. The more you handle your baby, the more your confidence will increase. Of course, the community midwife and then the health visitor and your own GP are there to advise you should you have any worries or problems. Ask your midwife or health visitor for a copy of the book which follows on from this one – *Birth to Five*.

COPING

'Everybody tells you how much having a baby's going to disrupt your life, your relationships – especially with your partner – but I didn't find that. Obviously, when you're both tired, nerves get frayed, but life's tons better with a baby than without.'

(A FATHER)

INVOLVING YOUR PARTNER

The more you can share your baby's care, the more you will both enjoy your baby. Your partner may not be able to breastfeed but he can help with bathing, changing and dressing as well as cuddling and playing. He may feel quite nervous of handling the baby and need encouragement. Be patient if he seems awkward at first.

HELP AT HOME

You'll probably need a lot of full-time help at first, not just with the chores, but also to give you emotional support. You're bound to feel up and down and to get easily tired in the early days. Many women want to have their partners with them so that they will have a chance to get to know the baby properly, as well as helping with the work. It also gives you some time to start adjusting to the changes in your life. If you're on your own, or your partner is unable to be with you, perhaps your mother or a close friend can be there. Even with help you will probably feel tired. Cut corners where you can.

- **Cut down on cleaning.** A bit of dust won't hurt.

- **Keep meals simple.** You need to eat well but this needn't involve a great deal of preparation and cooking.

- **Try to space visitors out.** Too many in a short time will be very tiring. If visitors do come, don't feel you have to tidy up or lay on a meal. Let them do things for you.

- **If you need extra help, ask.** Friends or neighbours will probably be very willing to do some shopping, for example.

LOOKING AFTER YOURSELF

REST

During the weeks or months that you are feeding your baby at night and your body is recovering from childbirth, finding time to catch up on rest is essential. It's tempting to use your baby's sleep times to catch up on chores, but try to have a sleep or a proper rest at least once a day.

PHYSICAL ACTIVITY

Continue with any postnatal exercises you were shown in hospital. You'll begin to benefit quite soon if you keep them up and they shouldn't be difficult to fit in during odd moments. Do your pelvic floor exercises (see page 16) – try doing ten sets of five tightenings a day. You can carry on with the stomach strengthening exercises (see page 16). Abdominal exercises to strengthen, firm and flatten your tummy should be done three or four times a day:

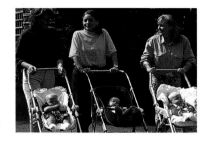

- lie on your back, with your feet on the floor, hip-width apart;

- press your back to the floor;

- put both hands on your thighs and curl your head and shoulders off the floor reaching towards your knees;

- breathe out as you go up, and in as you slowly come down;

- do 10 each time to start with, gradually increasing to 20, several times a day.

Besides these exercises, try to fit in a walk with your baby. A short walk in the fresh air will make you feel good.

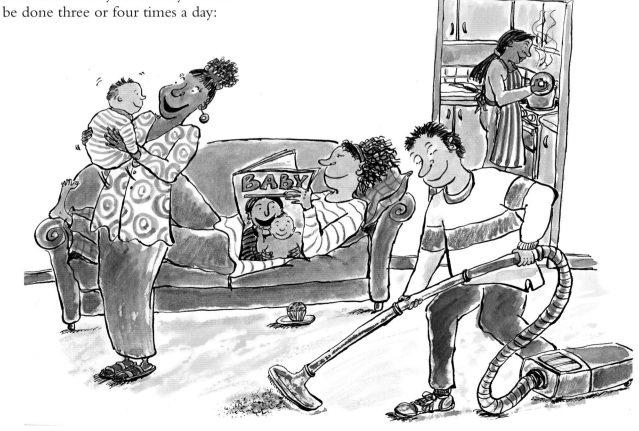

FOOD

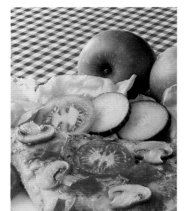

It's very important to continue to eat properly (see pages 8–10). If you want to lose weight, don't rush it. A varied diet without too many fatty foods will help you lose weight gradually. Try to make time to sit down, relax, enjoy your food and digest it properly. It doesn't have to be complicated. Try food like baked potatoes with baked beans and cheese, salads, pasta, French bread pizza, scrambled eggs or sardines on toast, for example, followed by fruit mixed with yoghurt or fromage frais.

A healthy diet is especially important if you're breastfeeding. Breastfeeding uses up a lot of energy. Some of the fat you put on in pregnancy will be used to help produce milk, but the rest of the nutrients will come from your diet. This means that you may be hungrier than usual. If you do need a snack, try having cheese or beans on toast, sandwiches, bowls of cereal or fruit. (See **Your diet when breastfeeding**, page 71).

YOUR RELATIONSHIPS

When you bring your new baby home all the relationships around you will start to shift and change. Your mother, for example, may find the change alarming and feel quite unsure of how much to get involved. You may find that she is trying to take you over or that she is so anxious to avoid bothering you that she doesn't help at all. Try to let the people close to you know clearly just how much you do want from them.

Your relationship with your partner will also change. It's very easy in those exhausting early weeks to just leave things to sort themselves out. Take care. You may wake up six months later to find that you haven't spent an hour alone together and have lost the easy knack of talking your problems through. You both need time alone, without the baby, to recharge your own batteries, and time together to keep in touch with each other.

Your relationship with the baby may not be easy either, particularly if you're not getting much sleep. Don't feel guilty if you sometimes feel resentful at the demands your baby makes, or if your feelings are not what you expected them to be. Talk to your midwife or health visitor if you're upset, but remember, many mothers do not feel instant love for their baby. They come to love them gradually over the weeks.

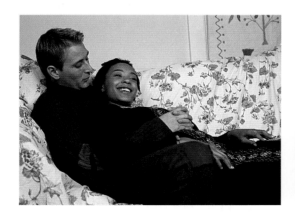

The 'baby blues' and postnatal depression

Up to 80% of mothers go through a patch of what is known as the 'baby blues', often about three or four days after the birth. You might feel very anxious about small things, for example, or mildly depressed or just keep bursting into tears, for no apparent reason.

Baby blues may be caused by hormone changes, tiredness, discomfort from sore stitches or sore breasts or even a feeling of anti-climax after all the excitement. Whatever the cause, you will usually find it only lasts a day or so. Have a good cry if you feel like it, and try to sleep if you can. The best help your partner or someone close can give is probably just to listen, give you a reassuring hug and look after the baby while you get some rest. If these feelings do not go away, it may be that you are simply not treating yourself very well. Take time out for treats, however small – a long lazy bath, your favourite food or visit a friend.

Around 10% of mothers slide into a depression which may be quite deep. They are taken over by a feeling of hopelessness. They may feel angry, but more often feel too exhausted to be angry or even to cope with the simplest tasks. If you feel like this you must get help. You should contact your GP or health visitor and explain how you are feeling. A partner or friend might contact them after talking to you about it. You can also contact the Association for Post-Natal Illness (see page 143) for more information.

Sex and contraception

There are no rules about when to start making love again. If you haven't had stitches you may be eager to share the extra love you feel with your partner. On the other hand, if you're tired and sore, sex may be the last thing you have in mind. Don't rush into it. If it hurts, it will be no pleasure. You may want to use a lubricating jelly the first time because hormone changes may make your vagina feel drier than usual.

It can take some time for the old feelings to come back but they will and, until they do, you may both feel happier finding other ways of being loving and close. If you have any worries, discuss them with your GP or health visitor.

It's possible for a woman to conceive even if she has not started her periods again or even if she is breastfeeding. Contraception should be discussed before you leave hospital and again when you go for your six-week postnatal check. In the meantime, you could talk to your midwife or health visitor when they visit you at home or you could go to your GP or family planning clinic.

The Family Planning Association (see page 143) publishes free leaflets about all methods of contraception.

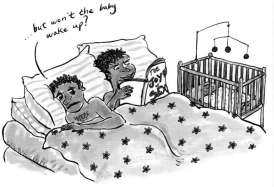

Possible methods of contraception

- **The condom** – *this may be the best and simplest choice for the early weeks after childbirth.*

- **The combined pill** – *if you're not breastfeeding, start taking this pill from the 21st day after delivery. If you start it later than the 21st day, it won't be reliable for the first seven days, so for this time you'll have to use some other form of contraceptive (like a condom) as well. Don't take this pill if you're breastfeeding as it reduces the milk flow.*

- **Progestogen-only pill** – *if you're breastfeeding, you may be offered a progestogen-only pill which will not affect your milk supply. This is also started on the 21st day after delivery and has to be taken at the same time every day. There's no evidence to suggest that this pill affects the baby in any way but, even so, some women prefer not to take any form of contraceptive pill while they are breastfeeding and use another form of contraception instead.*

- **Cap or diaphragm** – *these can be used six weeks after delivery. Your old one probably won't fit. Have a new one fitted at your postnatal check-up.*

- **IUD (intra-uterine device)** – *this can be fitted at your postnatal check-up when the womb is back to its normal size.*

THE POSTNATAL CHECK

You should have your postnatal check about six weeks after your baby's birth to make sure that you feel well and are recovering as you should from the birth. You may go to your own GP or may be asked to return to the hospital. It's a good opportunity to ask any questions and sort out any problems that are troubling you. You may like to make a list of questions to take along with you so that you don't forget what you want to ask. If you have had a Caesarean section you may like to ask if another one will be needed if you have another baby.

Routines do vary a little but the list below is probably what will be done.

- You may be **weighed**. You may be on the way to getting back to your normal weight again by now. Breastfeeding mothers tend to lose weight more quickly than those who are bottle feeding.

- Your **urine** may be tested to make sure your kidneys are working properly and that there is no infection.

- Your **blood pressure** may be checked.

- You may be offered an examination to see whether your **stitches** (if you had any) have healed, whether your **womb** is back to its normal size, and whether all the **muscles** used during labour and delivery are returning to normal. Tell the doctor if the examination is uncomfortable.

- Your **breasts** are unlikely to be examined unless you have a particular concern.

- The **cervical smear test** may be discussed if you haven't had one in the past three years (see page 55). This is usually delayed until three months after delivery.

- If you are **not immune to rubella** (German measles) and were not given an immunisation before you left hospital, you will be offered one now. You should not become pregnant for one month after this immunisation.

- The doctor will ask if you still have any **vaginal discharge** and whether you have had a **period** yet.

- There will be an opportunity to talk about **contraception**. If you have any worries over contraception or, indeed, any aspect of sex, now is a good time to discuss them. Tell your doctor if intercourse is painful.

- If you're feeling **very tired, low or depressed** make sure you tell the doctor about this.

- If you are having trouble holding your urine, or wind or are soiling yourself tell your doctor.

Your GP's surgery or health clinic will probably arrange for your baby's six-week check to be done at your postnatal check. If you go to the hospital, the baby's check will usually need to be arranged separately.

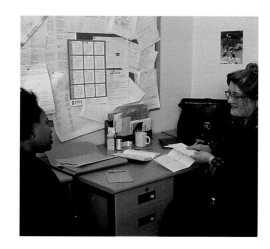

16 The early weeks: your baby

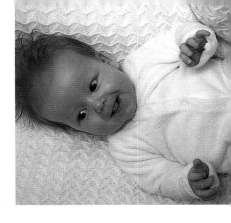

The baby's birth must be registered within six weeks from the date of birth at your nearest Registry Office. The address will be in the telephone book under the name of your local authority (in Northern Ireland, look under 'Registration of births, deaths and marriages'). If you are married, you or the father can register the birth. If you are not married you must go yourself, and if you want the father's name to appear on the birth certificate he must go with you.

REGISTERING THE BIRTH

If you live in a different district from the one where your baby was born, the registrar will take details from you and then send them to the district where the birth took place. You will then be sent the birth certificate. You cannot claim benefits or register your baby with a doctor until you have a birth certificate and a National Health Service number which will be issued at the same time.

CRYING

All babies cry. It's their way of saying that something isn't right. Sometimes you'll be able to find the reason for your baby's distress and deal with it. At other times all you can do is try to comfort or distract your baby. If it's not obvious why your baby is crying, think of possible reasons. Could it be:

- hunger?
- wet or dirty nappy?
- wind?
- colic?
- feeling hot, cold or uncomfortable?
- feeling tired and unable to sleep?
- feeling lonely and wanting company?
- feeling bored and wanting to play?

'I think there must be something there even before the birth. But it builds up as well. You know, it takes time to form a bond and over the months and years it grows stronger.'

'I think it has changed me. I think I've got a wider outlook on life now than I did before. And I can speak more openly to people. I can speak more freely. I'm more patient, too, whereas before I was very quick-tempered.'

It could be none of these things. Perhaps your baby simply feels overwhelmed and a bit frightened by all the new sights, sounds and sensations in the early weeks of life and needs time to adjust. Holding your baby close and talking in a soothing voice or singing softly will be reassuring.

Movement often helps to calm down crying. Gently sway or rock your baby or take your baby for a walk in the pram or baby carrier or even for a ride in a car. Sucking can

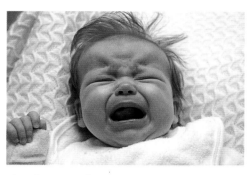

also be comforting. You can put your baby to your breast or give your baby a dummy if you wish. But if you do, make sure it is sterilised.

Do not dip the dummy in honey or sugar to make your baby suck – he or she will suck anyway. Using sugar will only encourage a craving for sweet things which are harmful to children's teeth.

Some babies do cry more than others and it's not really clear why. Don't blame yourself or your baby if he or she cries a lot. It can be very exhausting so try to get rest when

you can. Share soothing your baby with your partner. You could ask a friend or relative to take over for an hour from time to time, just to give you a break. If there's no one to turn to and you feel your patience is running out, leave your baby in the cot, put on some music to drown the noise, and go into another room for a few minutes. Make yourself a cup of tea, telephone a friend or find some other way to unwind. You'll cope better if you do.

Never shake your baby. Shaking makes a baby's head move violently. It can cause bleeding and damage the brain. Put the baby down safely in a cot or pram and calm yourself; don't be angry with the baby. If you feel you're having difficulties in coping with your baby's crying, talk to your midwife or health visitor. Or contact CRY-SIS (see page 143), who will put you in touch with other parents who've been in the same situation.

If your baby's crying sounds different or unusual, it may be the first sign of illness, particularly if the baby isn't feeding well or won't be comforted. If you think your baby is ill, contact your doctor immediately. In an emergency, if you cannot contact your doctor, take your baby to the nearest hospital Accident and Emergency Department.

SLEEPING

The amount babies sleep, even when they are very small, varies a lot. During the early weeks some babies sleep for most of the time between feeds. Others will be wide awake. As they grow older they begin to develop a pattern of waking and sleeping which changes as time goes by. Some babies need more sleep than others and at different times.

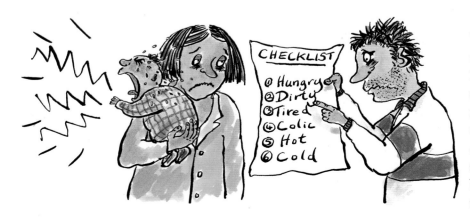

You'll gradually begin to recognise when your baby is ready for sleep and is likely to settle. Some babies settle better after a warm bath. Most sleep after a good feed. A baby who wants to sleep isn't likely to be disturbed by ordinary household noises, so there's no need to keep your whole home quiet while your baby sleeps. It will help you if your baby can get used to sleeping through a certain amount of noise.

See below for advice on sleeping positions.

REDUCING THE RISK OF COT DEATH

Sadly, we don't yet know why some babies die suddenly and for no apparent reason from what is called cot death or Sudden Infant Death Syndrome (SIDS). This section lists, in detail, all the advice we now have for reducing the risk of cot death as well as other dangers such as suffocation. There are three ways in which you can reduce the risk:

- **always put babies to sleep on their backs;**

- **avoid dressing your baby too warmly or overheating the room;**

- **do not smoke or allow others to smoke near your baby or the room your baby sleeps in.**

A SAFE PLACE TO SLEEP

Babies should always be put to sleep on their *backs* unless there is clear medical advice to do something different. Babies sleeping on their backs are *not* more likely to choke, and the risk of cot death is greatly increased for babies sleeping on

their fronts. Keep your baby's head uncovered and place your baby in the 'feet to foot' position to prevent your baby wriggling under the covers. Make the cot so that the covers reach no higher than your baby's shoulders.

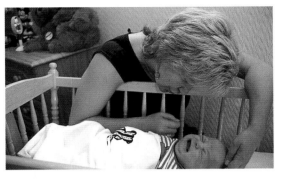

The 'feet to foot' position means that the baby's feet are right at the end of the cot to prevent the baby wriggling under the covers.

Ask your doctor or midwife for the leaflet, *Reduce the risk of cot death*, published by the Department of Health and Foundation for Study of Infant Death (FSID).

THE RIGHT TEMPERATURE

Small babies are not very good at controlling their own temperature. It's just as important to avoid getting too hot as it is to avoid getting chilled. Overheating is known to be a factor in cot death. Remember:

- if the room is warm enough for you to be comfortable wearing light clothing (16–20°C) then it is the right temperature for your baby;

- give your baby one light layer of clothing (or bedding) more than you are wearing. If the room is too hot for you, keep your baby's clothes or bed-covering light;

- don't use duvets (quilts) until your baby is a year old – they get too hot;

- keep your baby's head uncovered when inside (unless it's very cold) as babies need to lose heat from their heads and faces;

121

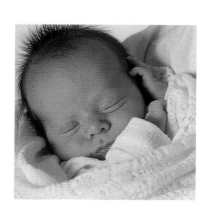

- never use a hot water bottle or electric blanket as babies have delicate skin which can scald easily;

- ill or feverish babies do *not* need any extra bedding – in fact, they usually need less;

- there has been some advice suggesting that it is unwise to have your baby in bed with you – there is no clear evidence of risk, but it would be wise not to have your baby in your bed if you have been drinking alcohol or have taken drugs which can cause drowsiness, and to be careful not to get the baby too hot;

- babies chill easily if it's cold, so wrap them up well when you go out, but **remember to take off the extra clothing when you come back inside**, even if you have to wake your baby to do it;

- avoid plastic sheets or bumpers, ribbons and bits of string from mobiles anywhere near your baby, who could get entangled in them;

- make sure there's no gap between the cot mattress and the sides of the cot which your baby's body could slip through;

- remove any loose plastic covering from the mattress which could come off and smother your baby.

You can protect your children by keeping their playing, sleeping and eating areas completely smoke free.

CLEAN AIR

Babies should not be exposed to tobacco smoke, either before birth or afterwards. If you, or anyone else who looks after your baby, smoke then don't smoke anywhere near the baby. Ask friends to smoke outside or before visiting you. It would be even better if everyone could make an effort to give up completely. Babies and young children who breathe in cigarette smoke are also more likely to get coughs, asthma and chest infections. For more advice on giving up smoking, see page 13.

COT MATTRESSES

There have been suggestions that toxic gases from fire-retardant materials found in some cot mattresses are another potential cause of cot death. However, a recent report examining this link found **no evidence** that cot mattresses contribute to cot death.

Following the advice given above will help to reduce the risk of cot death.

If your baby seems at all unwell, seek medical advice early and quickly.

Do remember that cot death is rare. Don't let worrying about cot death spoil the first precious months you have with your baby.

NAPPIES

Babies need their nappies changed fairly often, otherwise they become sore. Unless your baby is sleeping peacefully, always change a wet or dirty nappy and change your baby before or after each feed, whichever you prefer.

Organise the place where you change your baby so that everything you need is handy (see page 85). If you're using terry nappies, your midwife or your friends can show you different ways of folding them. Experiment to find out which method is easiest and best for you.

CHANGING NAPPIES

You need to clean your baby's bottom carefully each time you change a nappy to help prevent soreness.

- Take off the nappy. If it's dirty, wipe away the mess from your baby's bottom with tissues or cotton wool.

- Wash your baby's bottom and genitals with cotton wool and warm water and dry thoroughly. Or use baby lotion. For girls, wipe the bottom from front to back, away from the vagina so that germs won't infect the vagina or bladder. For boys, gently clean the foreskin of the penis, but don't pull it back; clean under the penis and the scrotum.

- You may want to use a cream such as zinc and castor oil cream which forms a waterproof coating to help protect the skin. Or you can just leave the skin clean and dry, especially with disposable nappies since cream may prevent them absorbing urine so well.

- Don't use baby powder as it can cause choking.

- If you're using a terry nappy, fold it and put a nappy liner inside, if you wish. Pin the corners of the nappy together with a proper nappy pin or clip which won't spring open.

- If you use disposable nappies, be very careful not to get cream on the tabs or they won't stick down.

- Put on, or tie on, the plastic pants, if you're using a terry nappy.

- Wash your hands.

NAPPY HYGIENE

Disposable nappies
If the nappy is dirty, flush the contents down the toilet. Roll up the nappy and re-tape it securely. Put it into a plastic bag kept only for this purpose. Fasten the bag and put it outside in your bin each day.

Terry nappies
- If the nappy is dirty, flush the contents down the toilet and rinse off the nappy in the flushing water.

- Have a plastic bucket (with a lid) ready filled with water and the right amount of nappy sanitising powder. Follow the instructions on the packet. Make sure you keep the nappy powder out of reach of small children.

- Put the dirty nappy to soak in the bucket.

- Wash each day's nappies in very hot water. Don't use enzyme (bio) washing powders as these may irritate your baby's skin. Rinse very thoroughly. Don't use fabric conditioners as they may also irritate the skin.

NAPPY RASH

Most babies get soreness or a nappy rash at some time, but some have extra sensitive skins. If you notice redness or spots, clean your baby very carefully and change nappies more frequently. Better still, give your baby time without a nappy and let the air get to the skin (keep a spare nappy handy to mop up). You will soon see the rash start to get better.

If your baby does have a rash, ask your midwife or health visitor about it. They may advise you to use a protective cream. If the rash seems

PUTTING ON A DISPOSABLE NAPPY

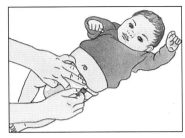

With disposables, the end with the sticky tapes goes under your baby's bottom. Fasten the tapes at the front.

PUTTING ON A TERRY NAPPY

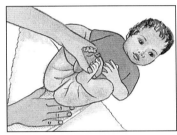

Lay your baby carefully on to a clean nappy and liner.

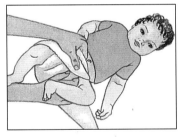

Bring the centre of the nappy between your baby's legs and then bring over the first side piece.

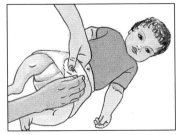

Bring over the second side piece and fasten all three pieces together with a nappy pin. Put on plastic pants over the top.

'You can't really explain, but it's a most wonderful thing to be a mum. To look after a baby and rear her, watching the different little things she does every day. It's just fantastic.'

to be painful and won't go away, see your health visitor or GP.

BABIES' STOOLS

Immediately after birth, and for the first few days, your baby is likely to pass a sticky black-green substance. This is called meconium and it is the waste that has collected in the bowels during the time spent in the womb.

As your baby begins to digest milk, the stools will change, probably becoming more yellow or orange. The colours can be quite bright. Breastfed babies have quite runny stools. Bottle-fed babies' stools are firmer and smell more.

Babies vary a lot in how often they pass stools. Some have a bowel movement at or around each feed; some can go for several days without having a movement. Either can be normal.

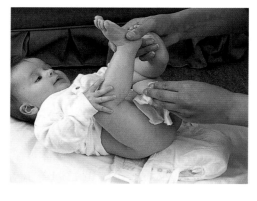

Most small babies strain and go red in the face, or even cry, when passing a stool. This is normal and doesn't mean they are constipated so long as the stools are soft. If you are worried that your baby may be constipated, mention this to your midwife or health visitor.

What you find in your baby's nappies will probably vary from day to day and usually there is no need to worry about how runny the stools are, for example. But if you notice a marked change of any kind in your baby's bowel movements, such as the stools becoming very frequent and watery or particularly smelly or if they change colour to become green, white or creamy, for example, then you should get advice from your doctor, midwife or health visitor. See **Babies with jaundice after two weeks**, page 113).

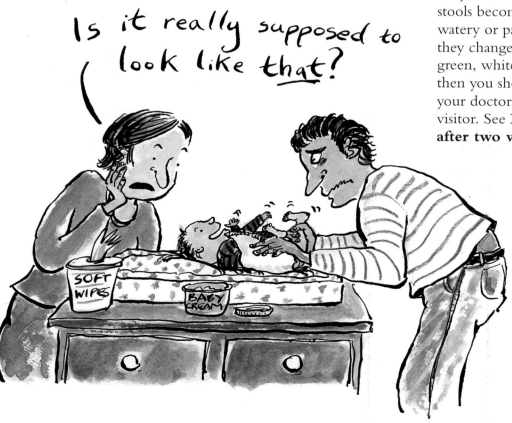

124

WASHING AND BATHING

WASHING

You don't need to bath your baby every day but you should wash your baby's face, neck, hands and bottom carefully each day. You can do this on your lap or on a changing mat. Choose a time when your baby is awake and contented and make sure the room is warm. You'll need a bowl of warm water, some cotton wool, a towel and a fresh nappy.

1 Take off your baby's clothes except for the vest and nappy. Wrap the baby in a towel.

2 Gently wipe round each eye, from the nose side outwards, using a fresh piece of cotton wool for each eye.

3 Using fresh, moist cotton wool again, wipe out each ear but don't clean inside the ears.

4 Wash the rest of your baby's face and neck with moist cotton wool and gently dry. Wash and dry your baby's hands in the same way.

5 Take off the nappy and wash your baby's genitals, again with cotton wool and warm water. Dry very carefully and put on a fresh nappy. In the first week or so, you should also clean round the navel each day. Your midwife will show you how.

BATHING

Bath your baby two or three times a week, or more often if your baby enjoys it. Don't bath straight after a feed or when your baby is hungry or sleepy. Make sure the room is warm and that you have everything you need ready in advance.

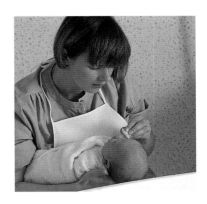

1 Check that the water is not too hot, just comfortably warm to your wrist or elbow.

2 Undress your baby, except for a nappy, and wrap snugly in a towel. Wash your baby's face with cotton wool and water as described above. Don't use soap on your baby's face.

3 Wash your baby's hair with baby soap or liquid, supporting the head over the baby bath or basin. Rinse carefully.

4 If you're using baby soap, unwrap your baby and soap all over, still on your lap so you have a firm grip. Take the nappy off at the last minute. If you're using baby bath liquid add it to the water at this stage.

5 Put your baby gently into the water. Using one hand for support, gently swish the water to wash your baby without splashing the face. You should *never* leave your baby alone in the water even for a few seconds.

6 Lift your baby out and pat dry with the towel. Dry carefully in all the creases. If your baby's skin is dry, gently massage in some baby oil. Your baby may enjoy this anyway.

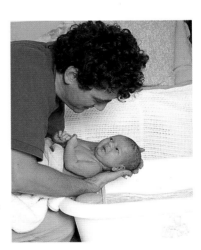

Never leave your baby alone in the bath.

If your baby seems frightened of the bath and cries, it may help to try bathing together. You may like to do this anyway. Make sure the water is only warm, not hot, and don't add anything to the water unless it's baby bath liquid.

ILLNESS

It's sometimes difficult to tell at first when a baby is ill but you may have a funny feeling that things aren't quite right. If you're at all worried, ask for help. You are not fussing. It's far better to be on the safe side, particularly with a very small baby. Trust your own judgement. You know your baby best.

VERY URGENT PROBLEMS

Sometimes there are more obvious signs that your baby is not well. Contact your doctor at once if your baby:

- makes jerky movements – this is a fit or convulsion;

- turns blue or very pale;

- has quick, difficult or grunting breathing, or unusual periods of breathing, for example if your baby breathes with pauses of over 20 seconds between breaths;

- is very hard to wake, or unusually drowsy, or doesn't seem to know you;

- develops a rash of red spots which do not fade and lose colour (blanch) when they are pressed. (See the 'Glass Test'.) This may be the rash of meningococcal septicaemia – an infection in the blood. There may not be any other symptoms.

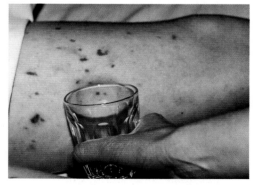

Your baby may need treatment very quickly. If you can't get hold of your GP at once, dial 999 for an ambulance or take your baby to the Accident and Emergency Department of your nearest hospital as quickly as possible.

PROBLEMS THAT COULD BE SERIOUS

- If your baby has a hoarse cough with noisy breathing, is wheezing, or cannot breathe through the nose.

- If your baby is unusually hot, cold or floppy.

- If your baby cries in an unusual way or for an unusually long time or seems to be in pain.

- If you notice any bleeding from the stump of the cord or from the nose, or any bruising.

- If your baby keeps refusing feeds.

- If your baby keeps vomiting a substantial part of feeds or has frequent watery diarrhoea. Vomiting and diarrhoea together may mean your baby is losing too much fluid and this may need prompt treatment.

- If your baby develops jaundice (looks yellow) when he or she is over a week old, or has jaundice which continues for over two weeks after birth (see page 113).

If you have seen your GP and your baby is not getting better or seems to be getting worse, tell your GP again the same day. If you become very worried and can't get hold of your GP or your GP can't get to you quickly enough, dial 999 for an ambulance or take your baby to the Accident and Emergency Department of the nearest hospital.

WHAT YOU CAN DO

- *You can contact your midwife or health visitor for advice. Keep their phone numbers where they can be reached easily.*

- *You can phone your GP. Your GP may be able to advise you over the phone or may suggest you bring your baby along to the next surgery. Most GPs will try to fit a young baby in without an appointment, although it may mean a wait in the surgery.*

If you're really worried about your baby, you should always phone your GP for help immediately, whatever the time of day or night. There will always be a doctor on duty even if it is not your own GP.

THE 'GLASS TEST'

Press the side or bottom of a glass firmly against the rash – you will be able to see if the rash fades and loses colour under the pressure. If it doesn't change colour, contact your GP immediately (see photo).

WHERE TO GET SUPPORT

Everyone needs advice or reassurance at some time or other when they are caring for a young baby, even if it's just to make sure that they are doing the right thing. Some problems just need talking over with someone. It's always better to ask for help than worry on your own. Do talk to your midwife or health visitor. As you grow more confident, you'll begin to trust your own judgement more. You will be able to decide which advice makes most sense for you and your baby and which suggestions you can safely ignore.

You will also want to talk to friends, relations or other mothers in a similar situation. You'll meet other mothers when you start taking your baby to the Child Health Clinic. Your health visitor will explain where this is and when you should go. The health visitor can also tell you about any mother and baby groups in the area. Or your local branch of the National Childbirth Trust (see page 141) or MAMA (Meet-A-Mum Association) (see page 142) may be able to put you in touch with other mothers nearby.

SUNSHINE

*In warm, sunny weather, **always** protect your baby from direct sunlight with a sunhat or sunshade. **Never** leave your baby in a place where he or she could become overheated.*

Remember too that a baby's skin burns easily, even in sun that would not affect your own. Use a high protection sunblock (at least protection factor 15+) to help protect your baby's skin from the sun.

ENJOYING YOUR BABY

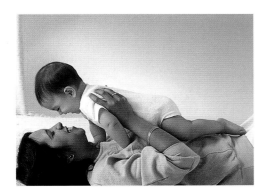

So far we have only talked about the things that have to be done to keep your baby warm, fed and safe. In the first weeks those things can grow to fill all the available time, but of course they're only a tiny part of what it means to be a parent. Every second that your baby is awake he or she is learning from you. Learning about what it feels like to be touched gently, about the sound of your voice and your very special smell, about what the world is like and whether it is a safe place to be and, above all, what it feels like to love and be loved.

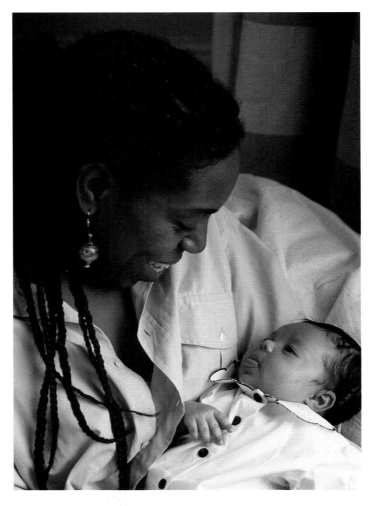

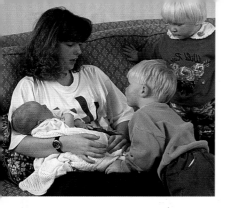

17 Thinking about the next baby?

As you hold your new baby in your arms, it may be impossible to imagine that you will ever have the energy to go through it all again. Or you may be eager to increase your family as soon as you can. Either way, this is the time to stop and think about how you and your partner can prepare for the next pregnancy. Nobody can guarantee that a baby will be born healthy. However, if you had a low birthweight baby or a baby with a disability or special needs, or a miscarriage or stillbirth, you may be particularly anxious to do everything you can to create the best possible circumstances for your next pregnancy. You'll want to talk to your doctor about this. If both parents are in good health at the moment of conception, that is the best start you can possibly give to a new life. There are a few other steps you can take as well.

DIFFICULTY CONCEIVING

It can take several months or more to conceive even if it happened really quickly the first time.

*If you're feeling very tired looking after the first baby, it may be that you are simply not making love at the right time. Re-read the section on **Conception** (pages 21–5) to remind yourself when you are most likely to succeed. If nothing happens after a few months, and you feel anxious about it, talk to your doctor or family planning clinic.*

FATHERS TOO

A bad diet, smoking, drinking and unhealthy working conditions can affect the quality of sperm and stop pregnancy from happening at all. Try to make your lifestyle as healthy as possible before you try to conceive.

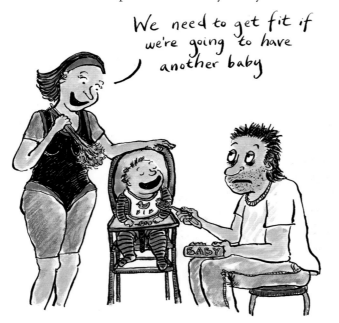

We need to get fit if we're going to have another baby

GETTING AND STAYING HEALTHY

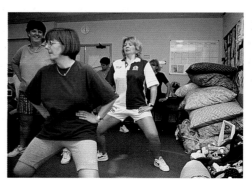

Re-read Chapter 1, **Your health in pregnancy,** about diet, smoking, alcohol and exercise. The advice is even more effective if you start well before the next baby is on the way. You will need to prepare for pregnancy by taking extra folic acid from the time you start trying to conceive right up until you're 12 weeks' pregnant. Choose foods that contain this important vitamin such as green, leafy vegetables and breakfast cereals and breads with added folic acid. (See symbol on this page.) To make sure you get enough, you should also take a 400 microgram (0.4 milligram) tablet every day. You can get these tablets from a supermarket or pharmacist. If you already have a baby with spina bifida, if you have coeliac disease or take anti-epileptic drugs, ask your GP for more advice, since you will need to take a bigger dose of folic acid.

THINGS TO THINK ABOUT

Here are some things that are worth doing before having your next baby.

Rubella (German measles)
Rubella can badly damage a baby during pregnancy. If you were not already immune you should have been offered immunisation immediately after your baby was born. Before trying for another baby, think about having a blood test to check that you are immune to rubella. The blood test will measure if you have enough protection (antibodies) against rubella. Women with low or uncertain levels of antibodies can be immunised again.

Long-term medication
If either of you has a chronic illness or disability and has to take long-term medication, talk to your doctor in advance of pregnancy about any possible effects on fertility or pregnancy. It may be possible to cut down the dosage.

Diabetes and epilepsy
If you have diabetes or epilepsy, talk to your doctor in advance.

Medicines and drugs
These may endanger your baby's health. Don't take any over-the-counter drugs at the time you hope to conceive without making sure

they are safe to take in pregnancy. Addictive drugs will affect your ability to conceive and, if you do conceive, are likely to damage your baby's health. See page 143 for organisations which can help you to stop.

Sexually transmitted infections (STIs)
STIs can affect your ability to conceive as well as affecting you. If there is any chance that either of you has been in contact with an STI, it's important to get it diagnosed and treated before starting another pregnancy. STIs, including HIV and hepatitis B, can be passed on through:

- sexual intercourse with an infected person, especially without using a condom, and some STIs can be transmitted during sex without penetration;

- HIV and hepatitis B can also be passed on by sharing equipment for injecting drugs.

If you're HIV positive, you could pass the virus on to your baby either in the womb, at birth, or by breastfeeding. About 15% of children born to mothers with the virus are likely to be infected (see box, page 54).

HAZARDS AT WORK

If you or your partner think there may be a risk involved in your work, talk to a union representative, your employer or personnel department. You have a legal right to know whether there is a definite risk. If there is a risk, ask if you can be moved to a safer job or, if this is not possible, find out whether wearing protective clothing, avoiding breathing in fumes and dust, and avoiding skin contact provide sufficient protection.

Foods carrying this mark have added folic acid.

VAGINAL BIRTH AFTER CAESAREAN SECTION

The majority of women who have had a Caesarean section are able to aim for a vaginal delivery for their next baby. This depends, however, on the reason for the first Caesarean section. Women who are thought to have a small pelvis, for example, may be advised to have a 'planned' (elective) Caesarean section next time. Your GP, or midwife, will be able to advise you. Most women who are advised to try for a vaginal delivery in subsequent pregnancies do have normal deliveries.

129

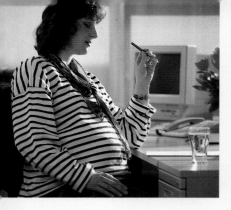

18 Rights and benefits

It's very important that you get help and advice as soon as you know that you're pregnant, to make sure that you know your rights and that you claim all the benefits to which you're entitled. Benefits have to be claimed on a lot of different forms, from many different offices, and the situation is always changing. The figures given here are accurate up to March 2000. Maternity rights are complex and sometimes change, so you should get further advice if you are unsure. There are many voluntary organisations that are happy to help. Don't hesitate to ask for advice. If in doubt, get a second opinion. See the box on where to get advice.

WHERE TO GET ADVICE AND HELP

Working out what benefits and rights you are entitled to and making claims can be complicated. Get help if you need it.

You can go to your local social security office (look in the business numbers section of the phone book under 'Benefits Agency'; in Northern Ireland 'Social Security Agency'). Or go to your local Citizens' Advice Bureau or other advice centre (see page 141). Social security offices can be very busy and an advice centre is often the best place to go. Citizens advice bureaux, law centres and other advice agencies will also be able to advise you about your rights at work.

Some local authorities have welfare officers. Phone your social services department (in Northern Ireland, local Health and Social Services Trust) and ask.

Some voluntary organisations offer information and advice on benefits and rights at work, for example, the National Council for One Parent Families and the Maternity Alliance (see pages 141 and 142).

If you are a member of a trade union, your staff representative or local office should be able to advise you on your maternity rights at work. The Equal Opportunities Commission can advise you if your problem is to do with sex discrimination (see page 141).

BENEFITS FOR ALL

Prescriptions and NHS dental treatment are free while you are pregnant and for 12 months after you have given birth. Your child also gets free prescriptions until age 16. To claim for prescriptions, ask your doctor or midwife for form FW8 and send it to your Health Authority (in Northern Ireland, Central Services Agency). You will be sent an exemption certificate which lasts until a year after your due date. To claim after your baby is born (if you didn't claim when you were pregnant) fill in form A in leaflet P11 *NHS Prescriptions* which you can get from your doctor or social security office (Benefits Agency). To claim for dental treatment, tick a box on a form provided by the dentist or show your exemption certificate (see above).

CHILD BENEFIT

What is it?
A tax-free benefit to help parents with the cost of caring for their children. It is payable for each child from birth until at least age 16.

Who gets it?
Every mother, but you must generally have been living in the United Kingdom for at least six months.

How much is it?
For your first child, £14.40 a week . (If you are a single parent claiming before June 1998 you get £17.10 a week for your first child.) For other children you get £9.60 a week per child.

IF YOUR INCOME IS LOW

How do I claim?

You may get a claim pack inside the Bounty Pack, which most new mothers are given in hospital. You can also get a claim pack from your social security office or post office (also General Registrar's office in Northern Ireland). Fill in the forms and send them with the baby's birth certificate to the Child Benefit Centre (Child Benefit Office in Northern Ireland). You will be given the birth certificate free when you register the birth. It will be returned to you. Child Benefit can be paid directly into your bank account or by a book of orders which you cash at the post office. It is usually paid every four weeks in arrears but single parents and families on low incomes can choose to be paid weekly. You should start to claim Child Benefit within one month of your baby's birth, otherwise you will lose some of the benefit.

Anything else?

Child Benefit can help to protect your State Retirement Pension if you stay at home to look after your child. For every complete year that you get Child Benefit but you don't pay enough National Insurance to count towards the basic pension, you automatically get 'Home Responsibilities Protection' which means that the year *will* be credited as counting towards your pension.

INCOME-BASED JOBSEEKER'S ALLOWANCE (JSA) AND INCOME SUPPORT

What are they?

Payments for people who are not in work and do not have enough to live on. If your family income falls below a set level the benefit will 'top it up'. This means you may be able to get income-based JSA or Income Support even if you are already getting Statutory Maternity Pay, Maternity Allowance, Incapacity Benefit or some income from part-time work.

Who gets them?

You can claim income-based JSA if you are 18 or over, *and* unemployed or working for less than 16 hours a week, *and* you are actively seeking work. If you are 16 or 17 years old you can claim JSA once your baby is born (but if you're single it's better to claim Income Support), or earlier if you face severe hardship.

You can claim Income Support if you are 16 or over, *and* either you're pregnant and incapable of work, *or* you're pregnant and within the period of 11 weeks before the baby is due until 7 weeks after the baby is born, *or* you're a lone parent. You must be unemployed or working for less than 16 hours a week. You do not have to be available for work.

You cannot claim income-based JSA or Income Support if you have a partner who works for 24 hours or more a week or if you have savings of more than £8000.

How much is it?

It depends on your age and the size of your family and what other income is coming in. If you're under 25 or have more than £3000 in savings you get a lower rate. If you're claiming during pregnancy you should let the social security office know as soon as the baby is born as your benefit will go up.

For example, if you are a single parent aged 18 or over with one baby and no savings, Income Support would top your income up to £85.50 per week. If you are in a couple aged 18 or over with one baby and no savings and you qualify for income-based JSA, the benefit would top your income up to £114.75 per week.

How do I claim?

Claim JSA by going to the Jobcentre in person (or by post if you live too far from the Jobcentre). In Northern Ireland claim JSA at your local social security office. Claim Income Support on form A1 which you can get from a social security office or post office. Return it to your social security office. The benefits are paid directly into your bank account or by Giro or by a book of orders which you cash at the post office. If you are claiming JSA you will have to go to the Jobcentre (Social Security Office in Northern Ireland) every fortnight to 'sign on' to show that you are available for work. If you are claiming Income Support you do not need to 'sign on'.

Anything else?

If you get Income Support or income-based JSA you can claim other benefits like a £100 Maternity Payment, free milk and vitamins, help with fares to hospital, Housing Benefit and Council Tax Benefit. You may be able to get help with mortgage interest payments.

FAMILY CREDIT

This will be replaced by the Working Families Tax Credit in October 1999.

What is it?

A tax-free weekly benefit for working parents on low pay.

Who gets it?

Families (including one-parent families) with at least one child where one parent works 16 hours a week or more.

The more children you have and the older they get, the more you can earn and still get Family Credit.

On your Child Benefit letter of award or benefit book there is a 'personalised message' which tells you how much your family can earn and qualify for Family Credit.

How much is it?

It depends how many children you have, how old they are, and what your income is. As a rough guide, if you have one child you may get Family Credit if your family income (after tax) is less than about £170 a week, or less than about £185 a week if you or your partner work 30 or more hours per week. If you pay for a registered childcare provider to look after your child, you may be able to earn up to £100 more and still get Family Credit. You cannot get Family Credit if you have savings of more than £8000, and you get less money if you have savings of over £3000.

How do I claim?

Claim on form FC1 which you can get from your social security office or a post office. You cannot claim before the birth of your first child. Family Credit normally lasts for 26 weeks and stays the same even if your circumstances change, so you may want to take advice about the best time to apply. Family Credit is paid straight into a bank account every four weeks or by a book of orders which you cash at the post office.

Anything else?

If you get Family Credit you can also claim a £100 Maternity Payment, help with fares to hospital and reduced-price formula milk. You may be able to get Housing Benefit and Council Tax Benefit.

£100 MATERNITY PAYMENT FROM THE SOCIAL FUND

This will be replaced by a £200 Sure Start Maternity Payment in April 2000.

What is it?

A one-off lump sum payment (a grant not a loan) to help buy things for a new baby.

Who gets it?

Pregnant women and new parents who are getting income-based JSA, Income Support, Family Credit or Disability Working Allowance.

How much is it?

A sum of £100 for each baby. If you have more than £500 in savings the payment will be reduced. For every £1 of savings over £500, £1 will be deducted.

How do I claim?

Claim using form SF100 which you can get from your social security office. You can claim any time from 11 weeks before the birth to 3 months after. If you can't get income-based JSA, Income Support or Family Credit until after your baby is born, claim the Maternity Payment before your baby is three months old. If you are claiming before the baby is born, send your maternity certificate, form MAT B1 (which you get from your GP or midwife when you're about 26 weeks' pregnant). If you're claiming after the birth, send the baby's birth certificate. It will be returned to you.

Anything else?

You can claim a Maternity Payment if you adopt a baby under a year old and you get one of the qualifying benefits. You must apply within three months of the adoption order.

SOCIAL FUND LOANS

The Social Fund can also provide interest-free loans to people in need. These loans are not a right and only limited money is available. The loan has to be repaid at a set amount per week (the amount depends on the size of the loan and your income and other debts). If your income is low and you need money urgently in a crisis, you may be able to get a Crisis Loan. If you

have been receiving income-based JSA or Income Support for at least 26 weeks and you need something essential that you can't afford to buy, you may be able to get a Budgeting Loan.

The Social Fund can also provide Community Care Grants to families receiving income-based JSA or Income Support in certain circumstances, such as to help pay fares to visit a mother and baby in hospital or to help a family under exceptional pressure. Grants do not have to be repaid.

HOUSING BENEFIT – HELP WITH YOUR RENT
(in Northern Ireland this will help with your rent and/or rates)

What is it?

Housing Benefit will help you pay your rent (in Northern Ireland rent and/or rates) if you're on JSA, Income Support, Family Credit or a low income. If you're a council tenant it will be paid to the council, and if you're a private tenant it will be paid either to you or direct to your landlord. In Northern Ireland it will be paid to the Northern Ireland Housing Executive if you're a Housing Executive tenant.

How much is it?

It depends on the rent you pay, average rents in your area, your income, savings, other benefits, your age and your family size. *It may not be the same amount as the rent you are actually paying.* You cannot get Housing Benefit if you have savings of more than £16,000 and the amount you get is reduced if you have savings of more than £3000.

How do I claim?

If you're getting income-based JSA or Income Support you will get a Housing Benefit claim form with your JSA/Income Support claim form. Otherwise get a form from your local council. In Northern Ireland if you're not claiming JSA/Income Support get an HB1 form from your Northern Ireland Housing Executive district office.

HELP WITH MORTGAGE INTEREST REPAYMENTS

Who gets it?

If you've got a mortgage and you're on income-based JSA or Income Support, you may be able to get help with your interest payments, although there is usually a waiting period during which you won't get any help.

How much is it?

You can only get help with interest payments (not repayment of capital or contributions to a linked PEP, endowment or insurance policy) and the amount is usually based on a standard average interest rate (which may not be the same as the interest you are paying). If you took out your mortgage before 2nd October 1995, you will get no help for 8 weeks, half of the allowable interest for the next 18 weeks and then all the allowable interest after that. If you took out your mortgage after 1st October 1995, you will get no help for 39 weeks and then all the allowable interest from the 40th week of your claim. If you claim benefit because of the death of your partner or because your partner has left you and you have at least one child under 16, you are treated as if you took out your mortgage before 2nd October 1995.

How do I claim?

Once you have claimed income-based JSA or Income Support, your social security office will automatically send you a form MI12 about your housing costs shortly before they become payable. You fill out part of the form and then send it on to your mortgage lender to fill out the rest. The money will either be paid to you as part of your income-based JSA/Income Support or directly to your mortgage lender. In Northern Ireland you should contact the Rate Collection Agency, Londonderry House, 21–27 Chichester Street, Belfast BT1 4UX.

Anything else?

Tell your mortgage lender as soon as you get into difficulties with your mortgage. If you are unable to meet your repayments you may be able to negotiate a temporary agreement for reduced repayments (e.g. during your maternity leave), and some mortgage agreements allow a few months 'repayment holiday' once during the life of the mortgage. If you have Mortgage Protection insurance contact your insurer immediately. Most insurance policies will pay out if you are receiving JSA or Income Support, but not if you are only receiving Statutory Maternity Pay or Maternity Allowance, so check carefully.

COUNCIL TAX BENEFIT
(Not applicable in Northern Ireland.)

What is it?

A benefit to help you pay your Council Tax if your income is low or you're getting JSA or Income Support.

Who gets it?

If your income is low or you're getting Family Credit, income-based JSA or Income Support, you may get Council Tax Benefit.

How much is it?

You may get all of your Council Tax paid or just part of it. It will depend on your income, savings, whether other adults live with you, and an assessment of your circumstances.

How do I claim?

If you're getting JSA or Income Support you will get a Council Tax claim form with your JSA/Income Support claim form. Otherwise get a form from your local council.

FREE MILK AND VITAMINS

What is it and who gets it?

You can get these free if you get **income-based JSA** or **Income Support**. You get **milk tokens** which can be used for one pint of milk a day for yourself while you're pregnant or breastfeeding, and also for your child up to age five. If your baby is under a year old, you can exchange his/her tokens for formula milk at Child Health Clinics and also from some pharmacies in Northern Ireland. You can exchange the tokens for normal milk with most shops and milkmen.

How do I claim?

To claim the tokens, tell your social security office you are pregnant and let them know the date the baby is due. If you collect your benefit from the post office you can collect your milk tokens at the same time, or they will be posted to you if your benefit is paid directly into your bank account.

You can also get free **vitamins** from antenatal and Child Health Clinics for yourself while you're pregnant or breastfeeding, and for your child up to age five. You do not need tokens but you may need to show proof that you are entitled (your benefit book or notice of award of benefit) and proof of your children's ages (such as the birth certificate or Child Benefit order book). Vitamin supplements should only be taken on the advice of your GP, midwife or health visitor.

REDUCED-PRICE MILK

If you get **Family Credit** and your child is under one you can buy formula milk at a reduced price from the Child Health Clinic and also from some pharmacies in Northern Ireland. Take your Family Credit book or letter of award to prove you're entitled. You may also have to prove your baby's age, for example, by showing the birth certificate or Child Benefit order book. At some clinics anyone can buy formula milk at a reduced price.

HELP WITH HOSPITAL FARES

If your family gets **income-based JSA, Income Support or Family Credit** you can get a refund for fares to and from the hospital (including visits for antenatal care). This can cover normal public transport fares, estimated petrol costs and taxi fares if there is no alternative. You claim at the hospital at the time you go there by showing proof that you get the benefit, or you can get a refund later (within three months) by filling in form HC5 which you can get from the hospital or social security office.

If your family has a **low income** you can also get help, but you first have to fill in form HC1 which you can get from your doctor, hospital or social security office.

Depending on how low your income is you will be given either certificate HC2 which means you qualify for free services or certificate HC3 which means that you qualify for some help. You show the certificate when you go to the hospital or claim later (within three months) on form HC5.

BENEFITS FOR WOMEN WHO WORK OR HAVE WORKED IN THE LAST FEW YEARS

MATERNITY ALLOWANCE

What is it?

A weekly allowance for women who can't get Statutory Maternity Pay (SMP). You can get Maternity Allowance if you

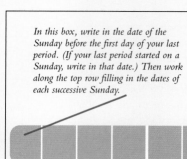

In this box, write in the date of the Sunday before the first day of your last period. (If your last period started on a Sunday, write in that date.) Then work along the top row filling in the dates of each successive Sunday.

THE TIMING OF YOUR RIGHTS AND BENEFITS IN PREGNANCY IS VERY COMPLICATED, SO USE THIS CHART AS A ROUGH GUIDE ONLY.

Write in the first day of your last period here. Then work along the row filling in the remaining boxes. Each box represents a week. Write in the dates week by week until you get to the date your baby is due.

are self-employed, if you gave up work or if you changed jobs during pregnancy.

Who gets it?

Women who can't get SMP but who have worked and paid full rate National Insurance contributions for at least 26 weeks out of the 66 weeks before the week in which the baby is due. If in doubt, claim. Your local social security office (in Northern Ireland, the Incapacity Benefits Branch, Castle Court, Royal Avenue, Belfast BT1 1SB) will work out whether or not you can get the benefit.

How much is it?

There are two rates. If you are self-employed or unemployed in the qualifying week (the 15th week before the expected week of childbirth), you get £51.70 per week. If you are employed in the qualifying week you get £59.55 per week. There are no deductions for tax or National Insurance.

When is it paid?

Maternity Allowance is paid for up to 18 weeks. It is only paid for weeks when you are not working. The earliest it can start is 11 weeks before the expected week of childbirth. If you are employed or self-employed you can choose when to start your Maternity Allowance in the same way as for SMP. However, if you are unemployed, your Maternity Allowance must start at week 11 before the week your baby is due.

How do I claim?

Fill in form MA1 (available from your Social Security Office or antenatal clinic) and send it to your local Benefits Agency (in Northern Ireland, the Incapacity Benefits Branch). You must also send: (1) your maternity certificate (form MAT B1) from your GP or midwife; (2) if you are employed, form SMP1 from your employer to show why you don't qualify for SMP. Send in form MA1 as soon as you are 26 weeks' pregnant. Don't put off sending it in because you are waiting for the MAT B1. You can send it later.

HAVE YOU CLAIMED EVERYTHING?

	Child Benefit	Free prescriptions	Free dental treatment	£100 Maternity Payment	Social Fund loans	Council Tax Benefit (not NI) & Housing Benefit	Help with mortgage	Free milk	Cheap baby milk	Free vitamins	Fares to hospital
Income-based JSA	✓	✓	✓	✓	✓	✓	✓	✓	✗	✓	✓
Income Support	✓	✓	✓	✓	✓	✓	✓	✓	✗	✓	✓
Family Credit	✓	✓	✓	✓	✗	✓	✗	✗	✓	✗	✓
Low income	✓	✓	✓	✗	✗	✓	✗	✗	✗	✗	✓

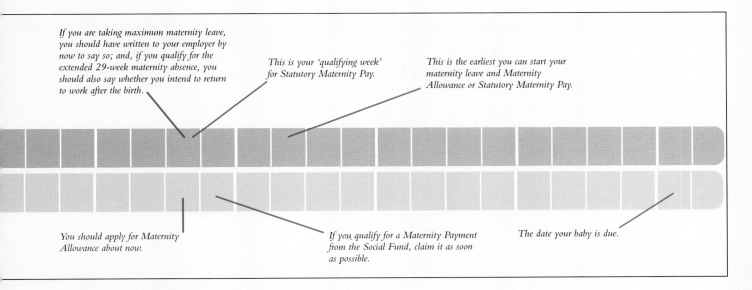

If you are taking maximum maternity leave, you should have written to your employer by now to say so; and, if you qualify for the extended 29-week maternity absence, you should also say whether you intend to return to work after the birth.

This is your 'qualifying week' for Statutory Maternity Pay.

This is the earliest you can start your maternity leave and Maternity Allowance or Statutory Maternity Pay.

You should apply for Maternity Allowance about now.

If you qualify for a Maternity Payment from the Social Fund, claim it as soon as possible.

The date your baby is due.

If you have not paid 26 weeks of National Insurance contributions by the time you are 26 weeks' pregnant, then you can decide to work later into your pregnancy. You should send off the MA1 form as soon as you have made up the 26 weeks of contributions. Maternity Allowance is paid by a book of orders which you cash, or directly into your bank account.

INCAPACITY BENEFIT

What is it?
A weekly allowance which can be paid to women from the 6th week before the week the baby is due until two weeks after the baby is born.

Who gets it?
Women who can't get SMP or Maternity Allowance but who have enough National Insurance contributions in earlier tax years. If you paid National Insurance contributions during the last three years, claim. Your social security office (Incapacity Benefits Branch in Northern Ireland) will work out whether you can get the benefit.

How much is it?
It is £50.35 per week. There are no deductions for tax or National Insurance. You won't get Incapacity Benefit for any week that you work.

How do I claim?
Make a claim for Maternity Allowance using form MA1 which you can get from your social security office or antenatal clinic. You have to send your maternity certificate, form MAT B1 (which you get from your doctor or midwife when you are about 26 weeks' pregnant) with your claim. You don't need to send in a sick note from your doctor. If you're not entitled to Maternity Allowance, the social security office (in Northern Ireland, the Incapacity Benefits Branch) will check automatically to see if you can get Incapacity Benefit. It can be paid directly into your bank account or by a book of orders which you cash.

CONTRIBUTION-BASED JOBSEEKER'S ALLOWANCE (JSA)

What is it?
An allowance which lasts for up to 26 weeks for people who are unemployed or working less than 16 hours a week (it replaced the Unemployment Benefit).

Who gets it?
You get it if you have paid enough National Insurance contributions during the last two tax years that do not overlap the current calendar year. You have to be available for work for as many hours as your caring responsibilities permit and you have to be actively seeking work.

How much is it?
If you are under 18 you get £30.95 a week, if you are aged 18–24 you get £40.70 a week; if you are 25 or over you get £51.40 a week. Your partner's earnings are not taken into account but, if you are in part-time work, your earnings are.

How do I claim?
Claim by going to the Jobcentre (Social Security Office in Northern Ireland) in person (or by post if you live too far from the Jobcentre). The benefit is paid directly into your bank account or by Giro every two weeks or by a book of orders which you cash at the post office. You will have to go to the Jobcentre (Social Security Office in Northern Ireland) every fortnight to 'sign on' to show that you are available for work.

If I resign from my job and don't go back to work after maternity leave, can I claim anything?
You may be able to claim contribution-based JSA for up to six months. However, you will have to show that you had 'just cause' for voluntarily leaving your job. You also have to be available for work for as many hours a week as your caring responsibilities permit (and not less than 16). If you haven't paid enough National Insurance contributions you may be able to claim income-based JSA (see above) instead, depending on your personal circumstances. Apply in person at the Jobcentre.

If you are a single parent you may be able to claim Income Support (see above) once the baby is born. If you are in a couple and your partner has a low income, you may be able to claim Family Credit (see above).

EMPLOYMENT RIGHTS

As a working mother-to-be, you are entitled to maternity leave, protection against unfair dismissal for pregnancy-related reasons, and protection against any health and safety risks to you at work. You may also be entitled to claim SMP when you stop work to have your baby. (Changes to leave and pay announced by the government in spring 1999 will not take effect until 2000.)

The information in this section tells you what rights and benefits you can claim and how to go about it. Your union representative, employer, or personnel department will be able to tell you if your workplace has any extra maternity rights better than the minimum. You still have the same rights to maternity leave and pay if your baby is born alive but premature (even if it only lives for an instant), or if your baby is stillborn after week 24 of pregnancy.

MATERNITY PAY FROM WORK

STATUTORY MATERNITY PAY (SMP)

What is it?
A weekly payment for women employed during pregnancy. Your employers pay it to you and then they claim most of it back from the Inland Revenue because it is really a State benefit. *You can get it even if you don't plan to go back to work. You will not have to pay it back if you don't return to work.*

Who gets it?
- You must have worked for the same employer for at least 26 weeks by the end of the 15th week before the week your baby is due (the 'qualifying week'). To find out what your qualifying week is, look on a calendar for the Sunday before the day your baby is due (or the day your baby is due if that is a Sunday). *Not* counting that Sunday, count back 15 Sundays from there. Your 'qualifying week' begins on that Sunday. You must have worked for your employer for at least 26 weeks by the end of the qualifying week to get SMP.

- You must also still be in your job during this qualifying week (it doesn't matter if you are off sick, or on holiday).

- You must earn £66 per week (before tax) or more on average during the eight weeks (if you are paid weekly) or two months (if you are paid monthly) before the end of the qualifying week.

If you are not sure whether or not you will get SMP, ask anyway. Your employer will work out whether or not you should get it.

How much is it?
For the first six weeks you get 90% of your average pay. (The average is calculated from the pay you actually received in the eight weeks or two months before the last pay day before the end of your qualifying week.) After that you get the basic rate SMP which is £59.55 per week for up to 12 weeks.

You won't get SMP for any week that you work. So, if you qualify for only 14 weeks of maternity leave and you return to work at the end of the 14th week, you will lose the last four weeks of your 18 weeks of SMP.

When is it paid?
It is up to you to decide when you want to start your maternity leave and pay. It always starts on the Sunday after you go on maternity leave so, if your last day of work is a Friday or Saturday, it will start at once. Week 11 before the birth is the earliest it can start, but you can work right up to the day your baby is due if you want to, and not lose any SMP.

The only exception to this rule is if you have a pregnancy-related illness in the last six weeks of your pregnancy. In that case, you will not be entitled to receive sick pay and you will start your maternity leave and SMP automatically. If your illness is not pregnancy-related, you can claim sick pay and start your SMP when you had planned to.

Your employer will pay you your SMP. They will deduct any tax and National Insurance contributions owing. It should be paid weekly or monthly, in the same way as you are usually paid.

How do I get it?
Write to your employer at least 21 days before you plan to stop work, telling them the date you are going on leave and asking them to pay you SMP. You must also send them your maternity certificate (MAT B1 form) which your GP or midwife will give you when you are about six months' pregnant.

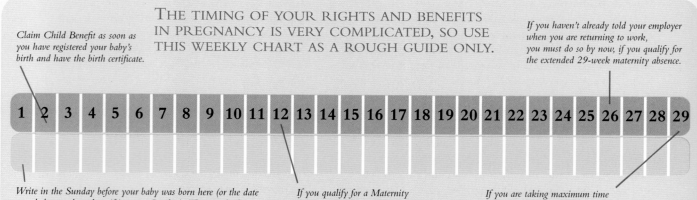

THE TIMING OF YOUR RIGHTS AND BENEFITS IN PREGNANCY IS VERY COMPLICATED, SO USE THIS WEEKLY CHART AS A ROUGH GUIDE ONLY.

Claim Child Benefit as soon as you have registered your baby's birth and have the birth certificate.

If you haven't already told your employer when you are returning to work, you must do so by now, if you qualify for the extended 29-week maternity absence.

1 2 3 4 5 6 7 8 9 10 11 12 13 14 15 16 17 18 19 20 21 22 23 24 25 26 27 28 29

Write in the Sunday before your baby was born here (or the date your baby was born here if it was a Sunday). Then work along the row filling in the remaining boxes. Each box represents a week.

If you qualify for a Maternity Payment from the Social Fund you must apply by now.

If you are taking maximum time off work, you must return to work before the end of this week.

MATERNITY LEAVE

FOURTEEN WEEKS MATERNITY LEAVE

Who gets it?

Every woman who is employed while she is pregnant is entitled to 14 weeks maternity leave, provided she gives her employer proper notice (see below). When you return to work it will be to exactly the same job. It doesn't matter how many hours you work per week and it doesn't matter how long you have worked for your employer, you still qualify for this right.

How do I get it?

Write to your employer *at least* 21 days before you start your maternity leave telling them (1) that you are pregnant and (2) the expected week of childbirth. You must also tell them (3) the date on which you intend to start your maternity leave (you only need to put this in writing if your employers ask for it). Finally you must, if your employers ask for it, (4) enclose a copy of your maternity certificate (form MAT B1) which your midwife or GP will give you when you are about six months' pregnant. If you cannot give 21 days' notice, for example, if you have to go into hospital unexpectedly, you must write to your employers as soon as you reasonably can.

When can I start it?

The earliest you can start your maternity leave is 11 weeks before the expected week of childbirth. It is for you to decide when you want to stop work. You can even work right up until the day of childbirth. The only exception to this rule is if you have a pregnancy-related illness/absence in the last six weeks of your pregnancy. If this happens, you may be bounced on to your maternity leave even if you are away from work for only one day. However, if you are ill only for a short time your employer may agree to let you start your maternity leave when you had planned. If your baby is born early, before the day you were planning to start your leave, then leave will start on the day of birth. If you are ill with a sickness that is not pregnancy-related, then you will be on sick leave and your maternity leave will start when you had planned.

What will I get while I'm away?

During the 14-week maternity leave period all your contractual rights (including holiday entitlement and benefits such as a company car) will continue as if you were not absent from work, except your normal pay. See Statutory Maternity Pay (above) for details of maternity pay.

What happens when I go back?

You do not need to give any notice of return if you are going back to work at the end of your 14-week maternity leave period (14 weeks from the day you began your leave). When you go back it will be to *exactly the same job.*

If you want to return to work early you must give your employers seven days' notice in writing of the date you will be returning. If you do not give this notice and just turn up at work before the end of the 14-week period, your employers can send you away for 7 days or until the end of your 14-week period, whichever is earlier. The law does not allow you to work for 2 weeks after childbirth

so, if your baby is born very late and your 14-week maternity leave period has run out, your maternity leave is extended by 2 weeks from the actual birth of your baby.

If you are unable to go back to work at the end of your 14-week maternity leave period because of sickness, you can remain off work for up to 4 weeks longer and still be protected from being unfairly dismissed if you have given your employer a medical certificate before the end of your maternity leave. If you are receiving SMP (see opposite) you will continue to receive it for these four weeks. If your employer has a contractual sick pay scheme you should get sick pay for these weeks.

EXTENDED MATERNITY ABSENCE

You may qualify for more time off after your baby is born – up to 29 weeks off from the week of childbirth.

Who gets it?

Women who have worked for the same employer for at least two years by the end of the 12th week before the week the baby is due. If you work in a firm which employs 5 or fewer people you do not have a clear right to return after 29 weeks even if you have the service, because your employer does not have to allow you to return to work if it is not reasonably practicable *either* to give you back your job *or* to give you suitable alternative work on terms and conditions which are not substantially less favourable to you. However, you still qualify for 14 weeks' maternity leave (see above) and you may well have a sex discrimination claim if your employer will not have you back. You should get further advice about your situation.

How do I get it?

As well as giving the notice for your 14 weeks' maternity leave, see (1)–(4) left, you must also (5) tell your employers that you intend to take extended maternity absence and return to work after the birth. (NB this does not mean you *have* to return – you can change your mind later). You must put this in writing at least 21 days before you start your leave, but you do not have to give a date for your return at this stage.

When can I start it and how long does it last?

The earliest you can leave work is the beginning of the 11th week before the *expected* week of childbirth. You can return to work at any time before the end of the 29th week from the *actual* week of childbirth. (Remember to count 29 weeks from the Sunday at the *beginning* of the week in which your baby is born – the week of birth is week 1).

What will I get while I'm away?

The first 14 weeks that you are away is ordinary maternity leave and so your contractual rights continue as set out under the Maternity Leave section above, but you do not get your normal pay: for details of maternity pay see under Statutory Maternity Pay (opposite). The rest of the time you are off is extended maternity absence and you should ask for your contractual rights to continue, but they may not necessarily do so.

What happens when I go back?

Your employers may write to you any time from 11 weeks after the start of your maternity leave asking you to confirm that you are going back to work. You must reply in writing *within* 14 days clearly saying that you are going back. This does not mean you have to go back: you can still change your mind later. It simply keeps open your option to return, otherwise you will lose that right. You don't have to give a date of return at this stage. If your employer doesn't write to you, you don't have to do anything. At least 21 days before you intend to return you *must write* to your employers giving notice of the exact date of your return. This is called your **notified date of return**. It cannot be later than the end of the 29th week.

When you return to work after extended maternity absence your employer must give you back the same job or, if that is not reasonably practicable, a suitable job on similar terms and conditions.

You cannot delay your return beyond the notified date of return except in certain situations.

- If you are ill you can delay going back for up to four weeks. You must let your employers know before the date on which you intended to return that you will be extending your leave because of sickness, and you must send in a medical certificate. If you are still ill after four weeks, you should seek further advice from the organisations listed on page 141.

- Your employers can also delay your return for up to four weeks. They must tell you the reason for the delay and give you a new date for your return. They don't have to pay your salary during these weeks.

- You may delay your return by agreement with your employer.

If you decide not to go back to work you should resign and give whatever notice is specified in your contract.

DISMISSAL OR UNFAIR TREATMENT

It is against the law for your employer to dismiss you or select you for redundancy for any reason connected with pregnancy, childbirth or maternity leave. It does not matter how long you have worked for your employer or how many hours a week you work.

If you are dismissed while you are pregnant or during your maternity leave, your employer must give you a written statement of the reasons.

If you are dismissed and you believe the reason is connected with your pregnancy, get advice from your trade union or local advice centre. You must put in your claim to the Employment Tribunal within three months of dismissal.

If you are sacked or are treated unfairly (e.g. having your pay cut) because you are pregnant or have had a baby, you may have a claim for sex discrimination. It doesn't matter how long you have worked for your employer. The law is complicated, so get advice. These claims also have to be made within three months.

HEALTH AND SAFETY RIGHTS

If you are pregnant, have given birth within the last six months or are breastfeeding, your employer must make sure that the kind of work you do and your working conditions will not put your health or your baby's health at risk. To get the full benefit of this legal protection you must notify your employer in writing that you are pregnant or have recently given birth or are breastfeeding.

Your employer is required to take the following steps:

- Carry out a risk assessment at your workplace.

- Do all that is reasonable to remove or reduce the risks found.

- Give you information on the risks and the protective measures.

- If the risks still remain, alter your working conditions or hours of work, if it is reasonable to do so and would avoid the risk.

- If this is not possible or would not avoid the risk, your employer must offer you a suitable alternative job.

- If this is not possible, your employer must suspend you on full pay for as long as is necessary to avoid the risks. If you have unreasonably refused alternative work offered by your employer you lose the right to full pay during your suspension.

- If you do night work and your doctor advises that you should stop for health and safety reasons, you have the right to transfer to day work or be suspended on full pay. You must provide a medical certificate.

You cannot be dismissed because a health and safety risk means that you are unable to do your normal job. If you are worried or are refused any of these rights you should consult your trade union or get legal advice.

TIME OFF FOR ANTENATAL CARE

All pregnant women have the right not to be unreasonably refused any time off work they need for antenatal care and to be paid for such time off. This means that you can take time off for your antenatal appointments, including time needed to travel to your clinic or GP, without loss of pay. All pregnant women have this right, whatever hours they work and however recently they started their job.

You should let your employer know when you need time off and how long you are likely to be away. For appointments after the first one, your employer can ask to see your appointment card and a certificate signed by your GP, midwife or health visitor, stating that you are pregnant.

Antenatal care includes parentcraft and relaxation classes so you should get paid for any time off you need to go to these classes. You may need a letter to show your employer from your GP, midwife or health visitor, saying these classes are part of your antenatal care.

If you are not paid or are refused time off you can make a claim to the Employment Tribunal within three months.

RETURN TO WORK ON CHILD-FRIENDLY HOURS

What are my rights?
If you want to change the way you work after having a baby, your employer must seriously consider your request. According to the Sex Discrimination Act, employers must have a good reason for refusing to let women work flexibly in order to look after their children.

Your employer will only be able to know if you can change the way you work by giving it a lot of thought. Refusing to even consider your request would probably be seen as unjustified if the matter went to an Employment Tribunal. So would having a policy of refusing part-time work. People often assume a job has to be done full-time or at certain fixed times of day. But, if you and your employer look carefully at your job, you may be able to work out a more child-friendly option – perhaps one that neither of you had considered before.

Does all this apply to me?
Employers must consider the request of any woman with children to work child-friendly hours. However, legal protection only applies if you would be disadvantaged by not being allowed to work the child-friendly hours you need to. In other words, you must have a good reason for asking to work differently, just as an employer must have a good reason for refusing.

Some good reasons for asking are:

- you can't find full-time childcare;

- you can't afford to pay for full-time childcare;

- you have to be there when your children come home from school perhaps because they have special needs;

- you are suffering from severe stress from working long hours (perhaps because your partner can't share the childcare).

What counts as a good reason for refusing?
Many of the arguments employers use do not count as justification at an Employment Tribunal. For example:

- there are no part-time vacancies (they should look at whether your own job could be done part-time or as a job-share);

- the job is too senior (the law applies to all women, no matter how senior);

- last-minute overtime is an essential part of the job (your employer should consider setting up a job-share, or an 'on call' rota);

- it is too expensive (costs are not usually any higher for part-timers);

- continuity is crucial (there are usually practical ways around this, like keeping good records and ways of communicating).

An employer probably would be justified in refusing flexible work if there were good business reasons and there was no alternative solution (e.g. if particular opening hours are necessary for business).

What do I do next?
You should sit down and discuss flexible working with your boss, someone from the personnel department and/or your union representative. If you are on maternity leave, you can write. You can look at the work you do now and consider how it could be done differently. If your employer agrees, they can't demote you, they must let you do the same job as before. You should be paid the same hourly rate as full-time staff and have the same contractual benefits such as holidays (but pro rata).

If you start to work part-time, you do not have the right to go back to full-time work later on, unless you have negotiated this with your employer.

If your employer refuses to let you work part-time you can take your case to an Employment Tribunal. You must apply for this within three months of your employer refusing your request to work part-time.

QUESTIONS WOMEN OFTEN ASK

When do I have to tell my employer I'm pregnant?

The latest time you can tell your employer is 21 days before you go on maternity leave. There is nothing to say that you have to tell your employer any earlier although it may be to your advantage – for example, your health and safety rights and your right to time off for antenatal care apply when your employer knows you are pregnant. Remember that the law protects you from being dismissed or discriminated against on the grounds of pregnancy once your employer knows you are pregnant.

Will I lose SMP if I work close to the birth?

It used to be true that you had to start your maternity leave at least six weeks before the expected week of childbirth or else you lost SMP. This has changed and now you do not lose SMP even if you choose to work right up to the birth.

How early can I leave work?

The earliest you can go on maternity leave is 11 weeks before the expected week of childbirth. So, if you work Monday to Friday, your last day of work could be the Friday of the 12th week before the expected week of childbirth.

Do I have to repay my SMP if I don't go back to work?

No – SMP (both the 90% of your pay and the £59.55 per week) is yours to keep whether you go back or not.

What happens if I say I want to return to work and I change my mind?

Giving 21 days' notice before you leave that you intend to return to work simply keeps your options open – it keeps open your *right* to return. Many women find it impossible to know before the birth how they will feel afterwards, so it is always a good idea to say you are coming back. If you decide later not to return you are simply resigning from your job in the normal way, so it is best to give your employer whatever notice is specified in your contract if you are leaving your job.

If I qualify for 18 weeks of SMP does that mean I get 18 weeks of leave?

Unfortunately no. Maternity leave and pay are two separate systems, so, if you do not have 2 years' service you only get 14 weeks' leave and pay, and you lose the last 4 weeks of SMP when you return to your job. However, it is always worth asking your employer whether they will give you 18 weeks leave – 14 weeks' is only the minimum. If they agree then you will get the 18 weeks' SMP.

YOUR MATERNITY RIGHTS

All employed women who are pregnant can claim:

- 14 weeks maternity leave;

- paid time off for antenatal classes;

- health and safety protection;

- the right not to be dismissed because of pregnancy.

Some women also have the right to:

- extended maternity absence up to 29 weeks from the week of birth;

- statutory maternity pay or maternity allowance.

The rights are the same for women whether they work part-time or full-time.

Mothers whose babies are stillborn after the 24th week of pregnancy can still qualify for all the rights described here.

The rights included here are all set down in law. Your workplace may have agreed maternity rights which are better than these so you should always check your contract or ask your union representative or the personnel department.

USEFUL ORGANISATIONS

Some of these organisations are large. Many are small. Some offer advice or information face to face or over the telephone. Others concentrate on providing useful leaflets or books. Many have local branches or can put you in touch with local groups or a local contact.

Where there are separate addresses in Wales and Northern Ireland, these are given. If the UK is not covered by one or more organisations the area covered is indicated by 'E' – England, 'W' – Wales, 'NI' – Northern Ireland. If you live in Wales you can contact Health Information Wales for further information.

Organisations marked * produce publications. When you write for information it's important to remember to enclose a large stamped addressed envelope for a reply. Many organisations are run by volunteers and nearly all have a very tight budget.

SUPPORT AND INFORMATION

ACAS (Advisory, Conciliation and Arbitration Service) (E, W)
Clifton House
83 Euston Road
London NW1 2RB
(020) 7396 5100
Advice on time off for antenatal care and on maternity rights and matters like unfair dismissal. For your nearest office, look in the phone book or ask at your local library or citizens advice bureau.*

Action on Pre-eclampsia (APEC)
31–33 College Road
Harrow
Middx HA1 1EJ
(020) 8427 4217 (helpline 10am–1pm)
National charity offering support and information about pre-eclampsia via its helpline and newsletters. Provides a befriender service.*

Active Birth Centre
25 Bickerton Road
London N19 5JT
(020) 7482 5554
Promotes a holistic approach to childbirth. Antenatal and postnatal classes (fee payable). Publishes list of UK active birth teachers.*

Association of Breastfeeding Mothers
PO Box 207
Bridgewater
Somerset TA6 7YT
(020) 7813 1481 (recorded information)
Telephone advice service for breastfeeding mothers. Local support groups.*

Association for Improvements in the Maternity Services (AIMS)
2 Bacon Lane
Hayling Island
Hampshire PO11 0DN
(01753) 652 781
Voluntary pressure group which aims for improvements in maternity services. Support and advice about parents' rights, complaints procedures and choices within maternity care, including home birth.*

British Diabetic Association
10 Queen Anne Street
London W1M 0BD
(020) 7323 1531

In Northern Ireland:
John Gibson House
257 Lisburn Road
Belfast BT9 7EN
(028) 9066 6646

In Wales:
BDA Wales
Plas Gwynt
Sophia Close
Cardiff CF1 9TD
(029) 2066 8276
Information and support for all diabetics.*

Caesarian Support Network
55 Cooil Drive
Douglas
Isle of Man IN2 2HF
(01624) 661 269 (after 6pm Mon–Fri and weekends)
Offers emotional support and practical advice to mothers who have had or may need a Caesarian delivery. Can put you in touch with a local mother who has undergone a Caesarian and understands the problems.*

Child
Charter House
43 St Leonards Road
Bexhill-on-Sea
E. Sussex TN40 1JA
(01424) 732631

In Wales:
Child Wales
202 Tyntyla Road
Ystrad Rhondda
(01443) 423500
Self-help organisation offering information and support to people coping with problems of infertility and childlessness. Telephone helplines for general problems and special helplines for specific problems like IVF, GIFT, ectopic pregnancies, miscarriages, stillbirths, endometriosis, polycystic ovaries and adoption. May be able to put you in touch with a local contact group.*

Child Poverty Action Group
94 White Lion Street
London N1 9PF
(020) 7837 7979

In Northern Ireland:
12 Queen Street
Londonderry BT48 7EG
(028) 7126 7777
Campaigns on behalf of low-income families. Provides advisers with information and advice for parents on benefits, housing, welfare rights, etc.*

Citizens advice bureaux
National Association of Citizens Advice Bureaux
Myddleton House
115–123 Pentonville Road
London N1 9LZ
(020) 7833 2181 (call for telephone number of your local office)

In Northern Ireland:
11 Upper Crescent
Belfast BT7 1NT
(028) 9073 9447
For advice on all benefits, housing, your rights generally, and many other problems. To find your local CAB look in the phone book or ask at your local library. There may also be other advice centres in your area offering similar help.

Community Health Councils
CHCs exist to help users of the NHS. They advise on where and how to get the service you need, and can help if you've got a complaint.

In Northern Ireland CHCs are called Health and Social Services Councils. For your local CHC, look in your phone book under the name of your district health authority or local Health and Social Services Council.

Commission for Racial Equality
10–12 Allington Street
London SW1E 5EH
(020) 7828 7022
Encourages good relations between people from different racial backgrounds, the elimination of racial discrimination and promotion of equal opportunities.

In Northern Ireland:
Community Relations Councils (CRCs)
Glendinning House
6 Murray Street
Belfast BT1 6DN
(028) 9043 9953

In Wales:
Race Equality First
Friary Centre
Cardiff CF10 3FA
(029) 2022 4097
Sometimes called Councils for Racial Equality or Community Relations Offices. They are concerned with race and community relations in their area and often know of local minority ethnic organisations and support groups. To find your CRC look in your phone book, ask at your town hall or local library, or contact the above.

Equal Opportunities Commission
Overseas House
Quay Street
Manchester M3 3HN
(0161) 833 9244

In Northern Ireland:
Chamber of Commerce House
22 Great Victoria Street
Belfast BT2 7BA
(028) 9024 2752
Information and advice on issues of discrimination and equal opportunities.*

Family Welfare Association
501–505 Kingsland Road
London E8 4AU
(020) 7254 6251
National charity providing free social work services and support for children and families. Provides financial support for families in need throughout the UK.*

Housing Rights Service (NI)
72 North Street
Belfast BT1 1LD
(028) 9024 5640
Helpline for people with housing problems. Offers advice and information on homelessness, housing debt, the private rented sector and Northern Ireland Housing Executive.

Independent Midwives Association
94 Auckland Road
Upper Norwood
London SE19 2DB
(020) 8406 3172
Free advice to women thinking about a home birth. Offers full care to women who book with them for home births. They also have their own birthing centres. Fees vary. Send an A5 SAE for information.*

Institute for Complementary Medicine
PO Box 194
London SE16 1QZ
(020) 7237 5165
Charity providing information on complementary medicine and referrals to qualified practitioners or helpful organisations.*

La Lèche League (Great Britain)
BM 3424
London WC1N 3XX
(020) 7242 1278
Help and information for women who want to breastfeed. Personal counselling. Local groups. Write with SAE for details of your nearest counsellor/group.*

Labour Relations Agency (NI)
2–8 Gordon Street
Belfast BT1 2LG
(028) 9032 1442
Advice on maternity rights in Northern Ireland.*

Life
Life House
Newbold Terrace
Leamington Spa
Warwickshire CV32 4EA
(01926) 421587
(01926) 311511 (national hotline 9am–9pm)
Charity offering information and advice on pregnancy, miscarriage, stillbirth and post-abortion counselling.

Local advice agencies
There may be a number of helpful local advice agencies in your district offering general advice on a range of topics, like benefits, debts and consumer problems, or specialising in one area such as law or housing. To find out what exists ask at your library or town hall.

Local health authorities
If you're new to an area they can give you a list of local doctors including those with a special interest in pregnancy and childbirth. If you have difficulty in finding a GP to take you on contact the LHA. Look in the phone book under the name of your local health authority/health board.

In Northern Ireland:
Contact your local Health and Social Services Board/Trust or the Central Services Agency for Health and Personal Social Services (CSA)
25 Adelaide Street
Belfast BT2 8FH
(028) 9032 4431

Maternity Alliance
45 Beech Street
London EC2P 2LX
(020) 7588 8583 (admin)
(020) 7588 8582 (advice line)
Information on all aspects of maternity care and rights. Advice on benefits, maternity rights at work.*

Minority Ethnic Health Liaison Project (NI)
Multi-Cultural Resource Centre (MCRC)
12 Upper Crescent
Belfast BT7 1NT
(028) 9024 4639
As part of MCRC, promotes two-way communication between minority ethnic groups and health service providers. Provides translation and interpreting services, multilingual materials and a reference library.

The Multiple Births Foundation
Queen Charlotte's and Chelsea Hospital
Goldhawk Road
London W6 0XG
(020) 8383 3519
For professional support of families with twins and multiple births.

National Association for Maternal and Child Welfare (NAMCW)
40–42 Osnaburgh Street
London NW1 3ND
(020) 7383 4117
Advice and courses on childcare and family life.*

National Childbirth Trust (NCT)
Alexandra House
Oldham Terrace
London W3 6NH
(020) 8992 8637
(9.30am–4.30pm Mon–Fri)
Information and support for mothers, including breastfeeding information, antenatal classes, postnatal groups. Write for details of your nearest branch and information pack.*

NSPCC (National Society for the Prevention of Cruelty to Children)
42 Curtain Road
London EC2A 3NH
(020) 7825 2500
0800 800500 (24-hour national helpline)

In Northern Ireland:
Jennymount Court
North Derby Street
Belfast BT15 3HN
(028) 9035 1135
Aims to prevent all forms of child abuse. If you're in need of help or know of anyone who needs help, look in the phone book for the number of your nearest NSPCC office.*

National Health Information Service England
Health Information Service Northern Ireland
Health Information Wales
0800 665544 (freephone 10am–5pm, minicom available)
A confidential information service on general health service matters and self-help groups.

Northern Ireland Housing Executive (NI)
2 Adelaide Street
Belfast BT2 8PB
(028) 9024 0588
Advice and information on all aspects of housing.

141

Patients' Association
PO Box 935
Harrow
Middx HA1 3YJ
(020) 8423 8999
Advice service for patients who
have difficulties with their doctor.*

Public libraries
Useful starting points for finding
out addresses of national and local
organisations. Librarians are usually
helpful in producing information or
pointing you in the right direction.

**RELATE: National Marriage
Guidance**
Herbert Gray College
Little Church Street
Rugby CV21 3AP
(01788) 573241

In Northern Ireland:
76 Dublin Road
Belfast BT2 7HP
(028) 9032 3454
Confidential counselling on
relationship problems of any
kind. To find your local branch
look under RELATE or Marriage
Guidance in the phone book or
contact the above addresses.

Shelter
88 Old Street
London EC1V 9HU
(020) 8881 3800

In Northern Ireland:
1–5 Coyles Place
Belfast BT7 1EL
(028) 9024 7752

In Wales:
25 Walter Road
Swansea SA1 5NN
(01792) 469400
Help for those who are homeless
and advice on any kind of housing
problem.*

Social security: local offices
For general advice on all social
security benefits, pensions
and National Insurance,
including maternity benefits
and Income Support and
income-based Jobseeker's
Allowance, telephone, write
or call in to your local social
security office. The address
will be in the phone book
under 'social security'.
Hours are usually 9.30am
to 3.30pm. In busy offices
there may be a very long wait
if you call in.

Social Services
A social worker at your
local social services office
will give you information on
topics including benefits,
housing, financial difficulties,
employment, relationship
problems, childcare and
useful organisations. Look up
social services in the phone
book under the name of your
local authority or, in Northern
Ireland, your Local Health and
Social Services Board/Trust or
ask at your local library. Phone,
write or call in. There may also
be a social worker based at the
hospital to whom you could
talk either during your antenatal
care or when you or your baby
are in hospital. Ask your midwife
or other hospital staff to put
you in contact.

**Twins and Multiple Births
Association (TAMBA)**
Harnott House
309 Chester Road
Ellesmere Port
Cheshire CH66 1QQ
(0870) 121 4000 or
(0151) 348 0020
(01732) 868000 (helpline
7pm–11pm Mon–Fri,
10am–11pm weekends)
Information and support for
parents of multiples. Network of
local Twins Clubs.*

ADDICTIVE DRUGS

Drugaid Caerphilly (W)
Substance Misuse Service
64–66 Cardiff Road
Caerphilly CF83 1JQ
Provides counselling and
information to drug/solvent
misusers and the general public.

**Narcotics Anonymous (UK
service)**
202 City Road
London EC1V 2PH
(020) 7251 4007
(020) 7730 0009 (helpline
10am–10pm)
Self-help organisations whose
members help each other to stay
clear of drugs. Write or phone
for information and the address
of your local group. Some groups
have a crèche.*

Or you can call the National
Drugs Helpline on Freephone
0800 776600. In Wales you can
also call Freephone 0800 371141
(Welsh). In Northern Ireland see
Dunlewey Substance Advice
Centre, Northlands and NICAS
under 'Alcohol'.

ALCOHOL

Alcoholics Anonymous (AA)
AA General Service Office
PO Box 1
Stonebow House
Stonebow
York YO1 7NJ
(01904) 644026

In Wales:
(South Wales)
(029) 2037 3939
(North Wales)
(01248) 716947
(Southwest Wales)
(01639) 644871

Network of independent self-help
groups whose members encourage
each other to stop drinking and
to stay off drink. First names only
are used to preserve anonymity.
For your nearest group look in
the phone book or contact the
AA General Service Office.*

Alcohol Concern
Waterbridge House
32–36 Loman Street
London SE1 0EE
(020) 7928 7377

In Wales:
Welsh Drug and Alcohol Unit
4th Floor
St David's House
Wood Street
Cardiff CF10 1ER
(029) 2066 7766
Can provide a list of organisations
offering help and advice.*

Drinkline
Alcohol Helpline
0800 917 8282

**Dunlewey Substance Advice
Centre (NI)**
226 Stewartstown Road
Belfast BT17 0LB
(028) 9061 1162
Help and counselling on alcohol,
drug and solvent abuse.

**Northern Ireland
Community Addiction
Service Ltd (NICAS) (NI)**
40 Elmwood Avenue
Belfast BT9 6AZ
(028) 9066 4434
Counselling, treatment, education,
information and training on dealing
with alcohol and drug addiction.

Northlands (NI)
13 Pump Street
Londonderry BT48 6JG
(028) 7126 3356
For treatment, training, education
and research about alcohol and
other drug-related problems.

CHILDCARE

Daycare Trust
Shoreditch Town Hall
Annexe
380 Old Street
London EC1V 9LT
(020) 7739 2866 (helpline
9.30am–5.30pm Mon–Fri)
Campaigns for the provision of
good childcare facilities. The
Daycare Trust gives information
on all aspects of childcare.*

**Mudiad Ysgolion
Meithrin/The National
Association of Welsh
Medium Nursery Schools
and Playgroups (W)**
145 Albany Road
Cardiff CF24 3NT
(029) 2048 5510
Help and advice on setting up
and running parent and toddler
groups and playgroups. Contact
with local playgroups.

**National Childminding
Association**
8 Masons Hill
Bromley BR2 9EY
(020) 8464 6164

In Northern Ireland:
17a Court Street
Newtownards BT23 7NX
(028) 9181 1015
An organisation for childminders,
childcare workers, parents, and
anyone with an interest in pre-
school care. Works to improve
status and conditions of
childminders and standards of
childcare.*

Pre-school Learning Alliance
69 King's Cross Road
London WC1X 9LL
(020) 7833 0991

In Northern Ireland:
NIPPA–The Early Years
Organisation
6c Wildflower Way
Apollo Road
Belfast BT12 6TA
(028) 9066 2825

In Wales:
Wales Pre-school Playgroups
Association
2A Chester Street
Wrexham LL13 8BD
(01978) 358195
Help and advice on setting up
and running parent and toddler
groups and playgroups. Contact
with local playgroups.

Working for Children
77 Holloway Road
London N7 8JZ
(020) 7700 0281
Advice and information for
employers, trade unions and
parents on developing childcare
at work.

COPING ALONE

Gingerbread
16–17 Clerkenwell Close
London EC1R 0AA
(020) 7336 8183

In Northern Ireland:
169 University Street
Belfast BT7 1HR
(028) 9023 1417

In Wales:
Room 1
Mansel House
99 Mansel Street
Swansea SA1 5UE
0800 018 4318 (freephone,
9am–4.30pm Mon–Fri)
Self-help association for one-
parent families. Local groups offer
support, friendship, information,
advice and practical help.

**Meet-a-mum Association
(MAMA)**
26 Avenue Road
South Norwood
London SE25 4DX
(020) 8771 5595
(020) 8768 0123 (helpline
7pm–10pm Mon–Fri)
Support for mothers suffering
from postnatal depression or
who feel lonely and isolated
looking after a child at home.
Will try to put you in touch with
another mother who has
experienced similar problems, or
with a group of mothers locally,
or help you to find ways of
meeting people. Write with SAE
for details of local groups.*

**National Council for One
Parent Families**
255 Kentish Town Road
London NW5 2LX
(020) 7267 1361
Free information for one-parent
families on financial, legal and
housing problems.*

Parents Advice Centre (NI)
Franklin House
12 Brunswick Street
Belfast BT2 7GE
(028) 9023 8800
(028) 7126 6663 (helpline)
(028) 8775 2900 (helpline)
(028) 2565 0099 (helpline)
Support, guidance and
counselling for parents with any
family difficulties.

Parents Anonymous
6–9 Manor Gardens
London N7 6LA
(020) 7263 8918
A 24-hour telephone answering
service Monday to Friday for
parents who feel they can't cope
or who feel they might abuse
their children.

DOMESTIC VIOLENCE

**Belfast Rape Crisis and
Sexual Abuse Centre (NI)**
29 Lower Donegall Street
Belfast BT1 2FG
(028) 9024 9696
Support and counselling to all
survivors of sexual abuse, rape
or incest.

NEXUS Institute (NI)
119 University Street
Belfast BT7 1HP
(028) 9032 6803
Provides a professional counselling
service to both males and females
over the age of 17 who have
been sexually abused or raped.

**NSPCC (National Society
for the Prevention of Cruelty
to Children)**
42 Curtain Road
London EC2A 3NH
(020) 7825 2500
0800 800500 (24-hour
national helpline)

In Northern Ireland:
Jennymount Court
North Derby Street
Belfast BT15 3HN
(028) 9035 1135
Aims to prevent all forms of child
abuse. If you're in need of help or
know of anyone who needs help,
look in the phone book for the
number of your nearest NSPCC
office.*

Rape Crisis
PO Box 69
London WC1X 9NJ
(020) 7837 1600 (24-hour
helpline)
Support and counselling for
women who have been raped.

Refuge
(0990) 995443 (24-hour
helpline)
Emergency accommodation and
advice for women and children
experiencing domestic violence
in London.

**Women's Aid Federation of
England**
PO Box 391
Bristol BS99 7WS
(01179) 444411
(administration)
(0345) 023468 (helpline
9am–5pm Mon–Fri)

In Northern Ireland:
129 University Street
Belfast BT7 1HP
(028) 9024 9041 (office)
(028) 9033 1818 (24-hour
helpline)

In Wales:
Welsh Women's Aid
4 Pound Place
Aberystwyth
Ceredigion SY23 1LX
(01970) 612748 (10am–4pm
Mon–Fri)
or
38–48 Crwys Road
Cardiff CF2 4NN
(029) 2039 0874
or
2nd Floor
26b Wellington Road
Rhyl
Clwyd LL18 1BN
(01745) 334767
Information, support and refuge for
abused women and their children.*

FAMILY PLANNING

**Brook Advisory Centres
(E & NI)**
165 Gray's Inn Road
London WC1X 8UD
0800 0185023 (helpline)
(020) 7708 1537
(administration)

In Northern Ireland:
29a North Street
Belfast BT1 1NA
(028) 9032 8866
Advice and practical help with contraception and pregnancy testing, advice on unplanned pregnancies and sexual counselling for young men and women. Free and confidential. For your nearest centre look in the local phone book or contact Brook Central Office.*

Family Planning Association
2–12 Pentonville Road
London N1 9FP
(020) 7837 5432

In Northern Ireland:
113 University Street
Belfast BT7 1HP
(028) 9032 5488

In Wales:
(North Wales)
Green House
Trevelyan Terrace
Bangor LL57 1AZ
(029) 2064 4034 (helpline)
(South Wales)
Ground Floor
Riverside House
31 Cathedral Road
Cardiff CF11 9HB
(029) 2064 4034
Information on all aspects of family planning and methods of contraception.*

Marie Stopes Clinic (E)
Marie Stopes House
108 Whitfield Street
London W1P 6BE
(020) 7388 0662

In Wales:
Marie Stopes Pregnancy One Call
PO Box 1343
Bristol BS99 3AJ
0800 716390
Registered charity providing family planning, women's health check-ups, male and female sterilisation, pregnancy testing, advice on unplanned pregnancies and sexual counselling for men and women. You don't need to be referred by your doctor, but you do need to book an appointment. A charge is made to cover costs. For centres in Manchester and Leeds look in the local phone book.*

HIV AND AIDS

AIDS Helpline (NI)
0800 137437 (7pm–10pm weekdays; 2pm–5pm Sat)

Body Positive
14 Greek Street
London W1V 5LE
(020) 7287 8010
0800 616212 (helpline, 7am–10pm Mon–Fri; 4pm–10pm Sat and Sun)

In Northern Ireland:
Room 308
Bryson House
28 Bedford Street
Belfast BT2 7FE
(028) 9023 5515 (2pm–4pm Tues–Fri)
Counselling services and support for women affected by HIV and AIDS, their family, partners and friends. For address and phone number of your local group phone the National AIDS Helpline or the above number.

National AIDS Helpline
0800 567123
National AIDS Helpline Language Line 0800 917 2227
For each of the languages listed below you can speak to an operator between 6pm and 10pm on the day shown.

At all other times this is a multi-language line and you can hear messages in each language.
Bengali — Monday
Urdu — Tuesday
Arabic — Wednesday
Gujerati — Thursday
Hindi — Friday
Punjabi — Saturday
Cantonese — Sunday

Positively Women
347–349 City Road
London EC1V 1LR
(020) 7713 0222 (helpline 10am–4.30pm Mon–Fri, Mon and Thurs 5pm–9pm)
(020) 7713 0444 (administration)
Information and practical and emotional support for women with a positive AIDS diagnosis or who have ARC or AIDS, including women who are pregnant or who have children. Support group.*

ILLNESS AND DISABILITY

Action for Sick Children (NAWCH) (E & NI)
300 Kingston Road
Wimbledon
London SW20 8LX
(020) 8542 4848

In Wales:
The Association for the Welfare of Children in Hospitals (AWCH Wales)
31 Penyrheol Drive
Sketty
Swansea SA2 9JT
(01792) 205227
Support for sick children and their families – helping parents to be with their child in hospital and informing families about hospital care.*

BLISS
17–21 Emerald Street
London WC1N 3QL
(020) 7831 9393
Parent support network providing emotional and practical support to the families of babies who need intensive or special care. Local branches.*

Contact a Family
170 Tottenham Court Road
London W1P 0HA
(020) 7383 3555
Links families of children with special needs through contact lines. All disabilities. Local parent support groups.*

Council for Disabled Children
Wakley Street
London EC1V 7QE
(020) 7843 6061
Information for parents and details of organisations offering help with particular disabilities.*

Disability Action (NI)
2 Annadale Avenue
Belfast BT7 3JH
(028) 9049 1011
Information and advice on physical disability and local organisations.

Disability Information Trust
Mary Marlborough Centre
Nuffield Orthopaedic Centre
Windmill Road
Headington
Oxford OX3 7LD
(01865) 227592 (answerphone)
Assesses and tests equipment for people with disabilities. Publishes information in series Equipment for Disabled People.

Disabled Living Foundation (DLF)
380–384 Harrow Road
London W9 2HU
(020) 7289 6111

In Northern Ireland:
Disabled Living Centre
Regional Disablement Services
Musgrave Park Hospital
Stockman's Lane
Belfast BT9 7JB
(028) 9066 9501 ext. 2708

In Wales:
Disability Wales
Llys Ifor
Crescent Road
Caerphilly CF83 1XL
(029) 2088 7325
Information and advice on all aspects of disability, especially equipment and daily living problems. Referral to other organisations for adults and children with disabilities.*

Genetic Interest Group (GIG)
Unit 4D
Leroy House
436 Essex Road
London N1 3QP
(020) 7704 3141
Umbrella body for support groups working with those affected by specific genetic disorders. Provides information for individuals at risk and their families about services available within the NHS and elsewhere. Can put you in touch with the relevant support groups.*

Northern Ireland Mother and Baby Appeal (NIMBA) (NI)
15 Stranmillis Road
Belfast BT9 5AF
(028) 9066 7166
A local charity offering support and advice to parents of premature, ill or disabled babies who need intensive or special care. A parents' support network is available throughout Northern Ireland, as well as practical services for parents.

Phab
Summit House
Wandle Road
Croydon CR0 1DF
(020) 8667 9443

In Northern Ireland:
Phab Northern Ireland
Mourne Villa
Knockbracken Healthcare Park
Belfast BT8 8BH
(028) 9079 6565

In Wales:
Phab Wales
2nd Floor St David's House
Wood Street
Cardiff CD1 1ES
(029) 2022 3677
Promotes integration between disabled and non-disabled people through social, leisure and educational activities.

LOSS AND BEREAVEMENT
(See also 'Child' under Support and information)

Antenatal Results and Choices (ARC)
73 Charlotte Street
London W1P 1LB
(020) 7631 0285 (helpline, 10am–6pm Mon–Fri)
Offers support and information to parents throughout antenatal testing, especially when a serious abnormality has been diagnosed and a choice has to be made about the termination of the pregnancy. Ongoing support given to those parents who decide on termination. Network of local contacts.

Compassionate Friends
53 North Street
Bristol BS3 1EN
(0117) 953 9639 (9.30am–5pm Mon–Fri)
An organisation of and for bereaved parents and families. Advice and support. Local groups.*

CRUSE Bereavement Care (E)
126 Sheen Road
Richmond
Surrey TW9 1UR
(020) 8940 4818 (Office)
(020) 8332 7227 (Helpline)

In Northern Ireland:
Piney Ridge
Knockbracken Healthcare Park
Saintfield Road
Belfast BT8 8BH
(028) 9079 2419

In Wales:
Old Bedw
Builth Wells
Powys LD2 3LQ
(01982) 560468
Offers help and counselling to bereaved people. Local groups

Foundation for the Study of Infant Deaths (Cot Death Research and Support)
14 Halkin Street
London SW1X 7DP
(020) 7235 0965 (administration)
(020) 7235 1721 (24-hour helpline)

In Northern Ireland:
Friends of the Foundation for the Study of Infant Deaths (NI)
7 Glenann Avenue
Belfast BT17 9AT
(028) 9062 2688

In Wales:
South Wales Scheme
12 Cotswold Avenue
Lisvane
Cardiff CF4 5TA
(029) 2076 4500
Support and information for parents bereaved by a sudden infant death and gives new parents advice on reducing risk of cot death.*

Miscarriage Association
c/o Clayton Hospital
Northgate
Wakefield
W. Yorks WF1 3JS
(01924) 200799
Information, advice and support for women who have had, or who are having, a miscarriage. Local contacts and groups.*

Stillbirth and Neonatal Death Society (SANDS)
28 Portland Place
London W1N 4DE
(020) 7436 5881 (10am–5pm Mon–Fri)
Information and a national network of support groups for bereaved parents.*

WIDWODS
c/o 60 Rocks Road
Uckfield
East Sussex TN22 2AX
(01825) 765084
Small support group of young widows aiming to provide practical and emotional support for those who experience the loss of a partner. Please include a stamped addressed envelope for written replies to any query.

SMOKING

ASH
16 Fitzhardinge Street
London W1H 9PL
(020) 7224 0743

In Wales:
374 Cowbridge Road East
Cardiff CF5 1JJ
(029) 2064 1101
(0345) 697500 (helpline)
Assists smokers wishing to stop and promotes non-smoking as the norm in society. Information and resource centre for the public.*

Quitline
(0800) 00 22 00

Quit (E)
Victory House
170 Tottenham Court Road
London W1P 0HA
(020) 7388 5775

In Wales:
Quitline in Wales
(0345) 697500
(9.30am–5.30pm Mon–Fri, recorded advice other times)
Advice on stopping smoking and details of local stop-smoking support services.

Ulster Cancer Foundation (NI)
40–42 Eglantine Avenue
Belfast BT9 6DX
(028) 9066 3281
Carries out cancer research and education programmes in Northern Ireland. Also provides information on the dangers of smoking and advice and support to smokers who want to quit.

SPECIALISED ORGANISATIONS

Association of Parents of Vaccine Damaged Children
78 Campden Road
Shipston-on-Stour
Warwickshire CV36 4DH
(01608) 661595
Advises parents on claiming vaccine damage payment.

Association for Spina Bifida and Hydrocephalus (ASBAH)
ASBAH House
42 Park Road
Peterborough PE1 2UQ
(01733) 555988

In Northern Ireland:
Graham House
Knockbracken Healthcare Park
Saintfield Road
Belfast BT8 8BH
(028) 9079 8878

In Wales:
(North Wales)
Canolfan yr Orsedd
Ffordd yr Orsedd
Llandudno
Conwy LL30 1LA
(01492) 878041 (10am–3pm
Tues, Wed, Fri)
(South Wales)
4 Lakeside
Barry
South Glamorgan CF62 6SS
(01446) 735714
Support for parents of children
with spina bifida and/or
hydrocephalus. Advice, practical
and financial help. Local groups.*

Cleft Lip and Palate
Association (CLAPA)
235–237 Finchley Road
London NW3 6LS
(020) 7431 0333
Voluntary organisation of parents
and professionals offering
support to families of babies
born with cleft lip and/or palate.
Feeding equipment available.
Local groups.*

Cystic Fibrosis Trust
11 London Road
Bromley BR1 1BY
(020) 8464 7211

In Northern Ireland:
178 Moyola Terrace
Portadown BT62 1BU
(028) 3833 4491

In Wales:
Cystic Fibrosis Research
Trust Wales (WCVA)
Llys Ifor
Crescent Road
Caerphilly CF8 1XL
(029) 2085 2751
Information and support for
parents of children with cystic
fibrosis and for people worried
about the possibility of passing
on the illness. Local groups.*

Down's Syndrome
Association (E & W)
155 Mitcham Road
London SW17 9PG
(020) 8682 4001 (10am–4pm
Tues–Thurs)

In Northern Ireland:
Graham House
Knockbracken Healthcare
Park
Saintfield Road
Belfast BT8 8BH
(028) 9070 4606

In Wales:
206 Whitchurch Road
Cardiff CF14 3NB
(029) 2052 2511
Information, advice, counselling
and support for parents of
children with Down's syndrome.
Local groups.*

Haemophilia Society
Chesterfield House
385 Euston Road
London NW1 3AU
(020) 7380 0600
(0800) 0186068 (helpline
9am–5pm Mon–Fri)

In Wales:
North Wales Group
54 Bastion Gardens
Prestatyn
Denbighshire LL19 7LU
(01745) 583910 ext 4092

In Northern Ireland:
Society House
6 Kilcoole Park
Belfast BT14 8LB
(028) 9072 9559
Information, advice and practical
help for families affected by
haemophilia. Some local groups.*

Jennifer Trust for Spinal
Muscular Atrophy
29b Avon House
New Broad Street
Stratford-upon-Avon CV37
6HW
(01789) 267520
Self-help group offering
information and support to
parents of children with the
disease. Can put you in touch
with other parents. Equipment
on loan.*

MENCAP (Royal Society for
Mentally Handicapped
Children and Adults)
MENCAP National Centre
123 Golden Lane
London EC1Y 0RT
(020) 7454 0454

In Northern Ireland:
Segal House
4 Annadale Avenue
Belfast BT7 3JH
(028) 9069 1351

In Wales:
31 Lambourne Crescent
Cardiff Business Park
Llanishen
Cardiff CF14 5GF
(029) 2074 7588
Information, support and advice
for parents of children with
learning disabilities. Local
branches.*

Meningitis Research
Foundation
13 High Street
Thornbury
Bristol BS35 2AE
(01454) 281811
(0808) 8003344 (24-hour
national helpline)

In Northern Ireland:
71a Botanic Avenue
Belfast BT7 1JL
(028) 9032 1283
Provides an in-depth support
network for families who have
undergone the trauma of a
bereavement and help and
information to families with
someone currently ill or
experiencing after-effects as a
result of meningitis and septicaemia.

Muscular Dystrophy Group
7–11 Prescott Place
London SW4 6BS
(020) 7720 8055
Support and advice through local
branches and a network of
Family Care Officers.

In Wales:
Muscular Dystrophy
Campaign
Institute of Medical Genetics
University Hospital of Wales
Heath Park
Cardiff CF4 4XW
(029) 2074 4021
Provides support for individuals
and families affected by
neuromacular conditions. .

National Society for
Phenylketonuria and Allied
Disorders
7 Lingley Lane
Wardley
Gateshead
Tyne and Wear N10 8BR
(0845 6039136)
Self-help organisation offering
information and support to
families affected by the disorder.
Newsletter.*

(NICOD) (NI)
Malcolm Sinclair House
31 Ulsterville Avenue
Belfast BT9 7AS
(028) 9066 6188
Offers advice and support to
parents of children with cerebral

palsy and related motor disorders.

Reach (The Association for
Children with Hand or Arm
Deficiency)
12 Wilson Way
Earls Barton
Northamptonshire NN6 0NZ
(01604) 811041
Information and support to
parents of children with hand or
arm problems. Can put you in
touch with individual families in a
similar situation or local groups.*

SENSE (National Deaf–Blind
and Rubella Association)
11–13 Clifton Terrace
Finsbury Park
London N4 3SR
(020) 7272 7774

In Wales:
SENSE Cymru
8 Forest View
Cimla
Neath SA11 3RS
(01639) 637115

In Northern Ireland:
The Manor House
51 Mallusk Road
Mallusk BT36 4RU
(028) 9083 3430
Advice and support for families
of deaf–blind and rubella-disabled
children.*

Sickle Cell Society
54 Station Road
Harlesden
London NW10 4UA
(020) 8961 7795/4006

In Wales:
Sickle Cell and Thalassaemia
Centre
Butetown Health Centre
Loudoun Square
Butetown
Cardiff CF11 5UZ
(029) 2047 1055
Information, advice, and
counselling for families affected
by sickle cell disease or trait.
Financial help when needed.*

Society for
Mucopolysacchoride Diseases
46 Woodside Road
Amersham
Buckinghamshire HP6 6AJ
(01494) 434156 (9am–5pm)
(01494) 762789
(answerphone)
Information and support for
families of children affected by
this and related disorders. Local
groups and regional clinics.

SCOPE
6 Market Road
London N7 9PW
(020) 7619 7100
(0800) 626216 (E and W
helpline 9am–9pm Mon–Fri,
2pm–6pm weekends)

In Wales:
SCOPE Cwmpas Cymru
Wales Partnership Area
Office
Brunel House
Ynys Bridge Court
Gwaelod-y-garth
Cardiff CF15 9SS
(029) 2081 3913
(029) 2081 0747 (Minicom)
Offers advice and support to
parents of children with cerebral
palsy.*

Tay Sachs and Allied
Diseases Association
c/o Postgraduate and
Research Centre
Royal Manchester Children's
Hospital
Pendlebury
Manchester M27 4HA

(0161) 794 4696 ext 2834
(answerphone)
Screening for carrier status
before and during pregnancy.
Information, counselling and
practical support to families
affected by these disorders.*

The Toxoplasmosis Trust
61–71 Collier Street
London N1 9BE
(020) 7713 0599 (helpline)
Information and advice for
pregnant women and support
and counselling for sufferers and
their families.

The UK Thalassaemia
Society
19 The Broadway
Southgate Circus
London N14 6PH
(020) 8882 0011
Information, and advice for
families affected by thalassaemia.*

SUPPORT FOR
STRESS AND
DEPRESSION
(See also Parents Advice Centre
and Parents Anonymous in the
Coping Alone Section)

Association for Post-Natal
Illness (APNI)
25 Jerdan Place
London SW6 1BE
(020) 7386 0868
Network of telephone and postal
volunteers who have suffered
from post-natal illness and offer
information, support and
encouragement on a one-to-one
basis. Send for information pack.

CRY-SIS (E, W, NI)
BM CRY-SIS
London WC1N 3XX
(020) 7404 5011 (8am–11pm)
Self-help and support for families
with excessively crying, sleepless
and demanding children. Write
for details with SAE.*

MIND (National Association
for Mental Health)
Granta House
15-19 Broadway
London E15 4BQ
(020) 3522 1754
0345 660 163 (Information
Line 9.30am–4.30pm
Mon–Fri)

In Northern Ireland:
NI Association for Mental
Health
Beacon House
80 University Street
Belfast BT7 1HE
(028) 9032 8474
Help for people with mental
illness. Also advice about coming
off antidepressants, tranquillisers,
etc. Local associations.

Parentline (E, W & NI)
Endway House
The Endway
Hadleigh
Essex SS7 2AN
(01702) 554782
0800 800 2222 (helpline,
9am–9pm weekdays,
2pm–6pm Sat)
A national helpline for anyone
parenting a child who may need
support, information or guidance.